Claude Annonier

Female Breast Examination

A Theoretical and Practical Guide to Breast Diagnosis

Translated from the French
by Richard Chambers

With 155 Figures and 6 Tables

Springer-Verlag
Berlin Heidelberg New York Tokyo

Dr. Claude Annonier

58, avenue Montaigne
F-75008 Paris

Translator

Richard Chambers

9bis, rue de la Grette
F-25000 Besançon

Translation of "L'exploration des seins de la femme –
Guide théorique et pratique de diagnostic sénologique"
 1st edition 1983

ISBN-13: 978-3-540-16302-2 e-ISBN-13: 978-3-642-82737-2
DOI: 10.1007/978-3-642-82737-2

Library of Congress Cataloging-in-Publication Data. Annonier, Claude. Female breast examination. Translation of: L'exploration des seins de la femme. Bibliography: p. Includes index. 1. Breast – Diseases – Diagnosis. I. Title. [DNLM: 1. Breast Diseases – diagnosis. WP 815 A615e] RG493.A5513 1986 618.1'9075 86-11914

Softcover reprint of the hardover 1st edition 1986

Bookbinding: Konrad Triltsch, Graphischer Betrieb, Würzburg
2121/3130-543210

Foreword

While radiology only reveals one aspect of the entire anatomical picture, a certain diagnostic precision can be attained by skillfully combining different techniques. The resulting images often uncover the hidden reality. This near perfection is most clearly seen – and is also most essential – in the study of the breast. One must remember that in the western world, one woman in fifteen develops breast cancer. It follows that the key to effective treatment is early and precise diagnosis. An understanding of the various breast tissues and of benign pathology is also indispensable in determining local risk.

How to achieve this goal of early and precise diagnosis is the problem addressed in this well-documented text demonstrating the considerable experience of Dr. Claude Annonier. A fresh look at the technical aspects and a complete clinical analysis together show the successes and limitations of modern methods and the need to combine different techniques in most cases. Evaluation of the various methods provides justification, if still needed, for the author's contention that mammography alone is insufficient. Progress in the field is making it possible to detect smaller and smaller lesions, whose malignancy cannot be determined without needle or surgical biopsy. More generally, the author underlines the necessity for complete cooperation between diagnostician and therapist. Follow-up for the "treated" breast is largely in the hands of the radiologist, who must, however, work together with other specialists. It is essential that he understand the endocrine, chemotherapeutic, radiotherapeutic, and surgical problems which may modify the results of his examinations.

As with many new techniques, breast imaging had its phase of unrealistic promises. It is currently going through a "sorting-out" period in which indications for the different methods are being defined.

This highly informative text will help to determine an overall diagnostic strategy. It demonstrates the necessity for adapting the strategy to each clinical situation and for bringing together experience and technique, diagnostician and therapist, in order to effect a cure.

PROFESSOR M. LAVAL-JEANTET

Contents

Introduction

Only a short time ago, breast examination could be summed up in just a few lines:

- All masses were to be biopsied and subject to frozen section examination. If carcinoma was diagnosed, treatment consisted of immediate and extensive removal.
- Any abnormality not associated with a mass (pain, infection, trauma) was treated in the same manner as it would be in any other soft tissue.

Progress in diagnosis and treatment for breast diseases have radically changed this conception for the benefit of our patients, a benefit which is only assured, however, if we adhere to the two fundamental qualities of the old conception: precision and coherence.

One of the characteristics of breast examination is that each new advance has been a divisive factor for medical personnel. Cure-all for some, fraud for others, it causes heated debate which confuses the practitioner and offers irrational temptation to those concerned.

Mammography was the first upheaval. While today almost universally accepted, it is certainly the method which encountered the greatest indifference, then hostility. In 1913, Salomon (Berlin) published a study showing the relationship between radiographs of surgical specimens and pathology. It was not until 1947 that Leborgne (Montevideo) and then in 1950 Gros (Strasbourg) indicated the future of mammary radiodiagnosis. Even then, mammography remained in the background while decisions continued to be based on clinical evidence.

Two developments challenged traditional ideas: From a diagnostic standpoint, the radiographic image improved considerably and new techniques became available: transillumination, thermography, ultrasonography, and needle biopsy. Noninvasive diagnosis was now possible. Nonmutilating, nonsurgical treatment of breast carcinoma also became possible. Thus, such noninvasive diagnosis of breast disease became both possible and desirable not only for malignant pathology but even more so for benign pathology.

Traditional rules mentioned above now became obsolete:

- A mass might not have to be removed.
- Biopsy may be necessary for a nonpalpable lesion detected by paraclinical methods.

There are certain risks when numerous techniques are involved. Safety requirements which today are joined by cost considerations demand that the actual capabilities of each technique be understood and that the role (or roles) of each be precisely defined: decision, examination, analysis.

The physician requesting an examination should be, if possible, the one to deal with the results. He knows (and makes known) the reason for the examination: screening, diagnosis, follow-up.

The physician who applies one or several examination techniques is usually the best professional judge of the quality of the results. But, his role differs depending on whether he is only responsible for one part of the examination or for the final analysis. In the former case, he should avoid making conclusions which might conflict with those of another technique. For example, a radiologist should not indicate the need for open biopsy when the film of a mass shows an opacity without specific signs. Ultrasonography might, in this case, demonstrate a cyst which could be insufflated or thermography could show strong hyperthermia contraindicating surgery, at least temporarily.

In the latter case, he must formulate a definite plan. If several possibilities seem reasonable, each one should be outlined, leaving the choice up to the decision-making physician, who in turn may have additional information which will influence his decision.

This distribution of roles is certainly flexible. A physician can easily assume several roles: decision-making, examining, and analyzing, providing none is overshadowed and providing he does not overstep his area of expertise without justified medical grounds. A good example is the radiologist, who needs no authorization, other than that of the patient, for cystography or galactography. Except for certain necessary therapeutic tests, however, it is not for him to prescribe treatment.

1 Sources of Information

1.1 History of the Disease

Use of a special form is recommended so that nothing will be forgotten and in order to quickly note and easily visualize the essentials (Fig. 1).

1.1.1 Chief Complaint

This is the initial indication, which may lead to detection of an abnormality during the examination. A symptom reported by the patient should always be taken into consideration even if not evident during the examination. The principal presenting symptoms, of which pain is the most frequent, are noted on the form.

1.1.2 Past Medical History

The form should mention all gynecologic and endocrine diseases or operations. It is also a good idea to note the date and conclusions of previous breast examinations.

The ob-gyn history completes this section:

- Age of menarche and duration of pubertal dysmenorrhea
- Age at each pregnancy (whether to term or not)
- Duration of nursing
- Puerperal mastitis
- Oral contraception: type, age, duration
- Age at menopause and duration of premenopause

1.1.3 Characteristics of the Menstrual Cycle

Regularity, rhythm, duration, premenstrual syndrome.

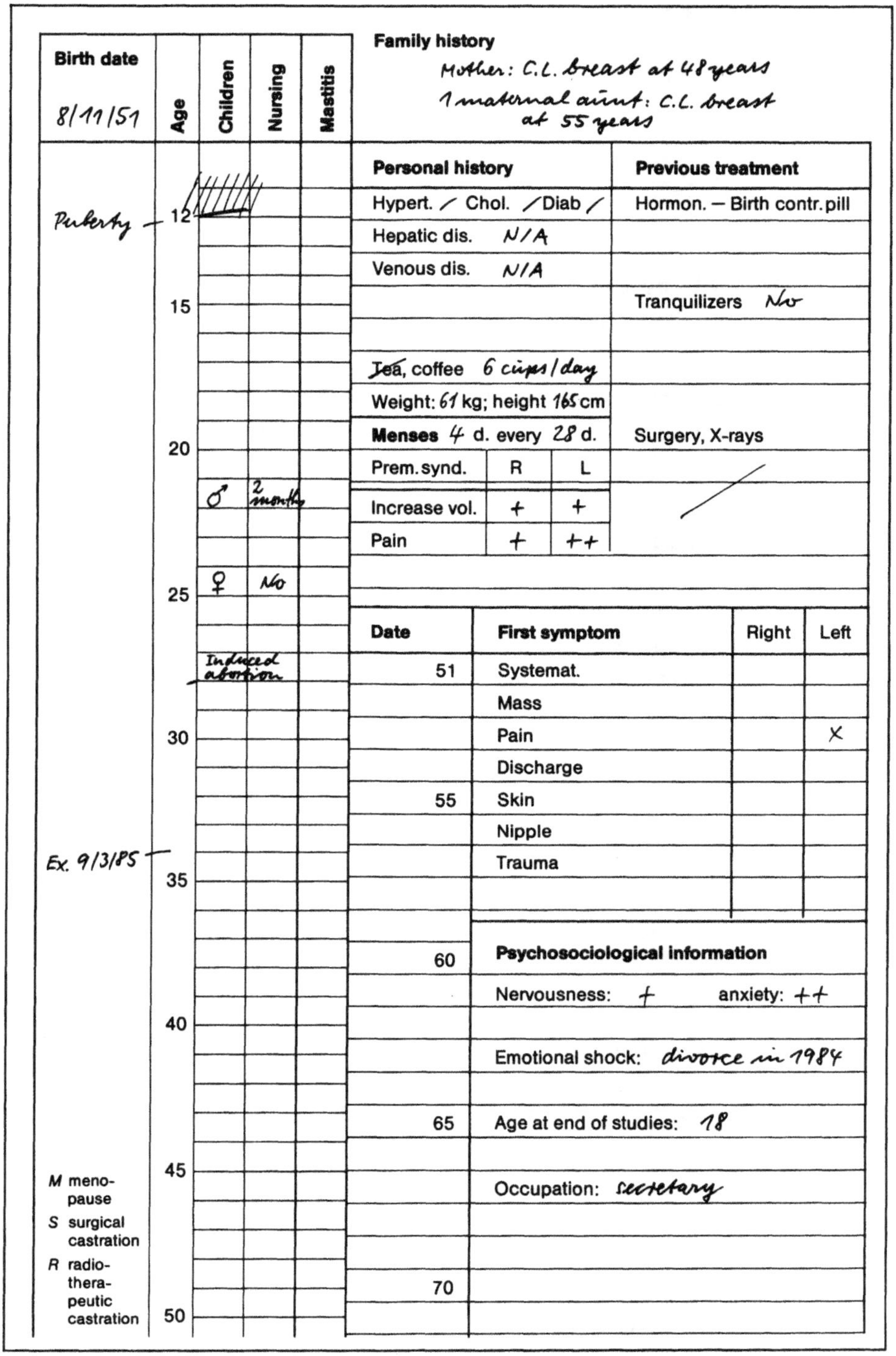

Birth date 8/11/51

Age	Children	Nursing	Mastitis
12 (Puberty)			
15			
20			
	♂	2 months	
25	♀	No	
	Induced abortion		
30			
35 (Ex. 9/3/85)			
40			
45			
50			

M menopause
S surgical castration
R radiotherapeutic castration

Family history
Mother: C.L. breast at 48 years
1 maternal aunt: C.L. breast at 55 years

Personal history			**Previous treatment**
Hypert. / Chol. / Diab /			Hormon. – Birth contr. pill
Hepatic dis. N/A			
Venous dis. N/A			
			Tranquilizers No
~~Tea~~, coffee 6 cups/day			
Weight: 61 kg; height 165 cm			
Menses 4 d. every 28 d.			Surgery, X-rays
Prem. synd.	R	L	/
Increase vol.	+	+	
Pain	+	++	

Date	First symptom	Right	Left
51	Systemat.		
	Mass		
	Pain		×
	Discharge		
55	Skin		
	Nipple		
	Trauma		

Date	**Psychosociological information**
60	Nervousness: + anxiety: ++
	Emotional shock: divorce in 1984
65	Age at end of studies: 18
	Occupation: secretary
70	

Fig. 1. History of the disease

1.1.4 Medical and Psychologic Background

- Chronic diseases, particularly arterial hypertension, hypercholesterolemia, diabetes
- Vascular disease
- Nervousness, anxiety
- Regular use of medications, particularly psychotropics and antihypertensives, tea and coffee consumption
- Height and weight

1.1.5 Social and Family Background

- Education (age at the end of studies)
- Profession
- Marital and family status
- Emotional trauma, recent change in status

1.1.6 Family History

While breast cancer of the mother or a sister should be noted, it is also important to note any breast cancer of more distant relatives and carcinoma of other organs. It is also useful to know the family history of any benign disease and the age of the mother when the patient was born.

Interpreting the History of the Disease

Several factors should be considered:
- Those which modify appearances observed during the different examinations: date of the menstrual cycle, endocrine abnormalities
- Those which may cause tissue scarring: trauma, operations
- Those which may affect the hypothalamic-hypophyseal-gonadal axis
- Those which are risk factors of breast cancer

Strong Point
Risk factors of cancer, nonmedical causes of functional disease

1.2 The Clinical Picture

1.2.1 Functional Signs

Since these are variably perceived, they are not necessarily presenting symptoms.

1.2.1.1 Pain

- Spontaneous or tenderness on compression
- Uni- or bilateral
- Radiating or radiating from the shoulder, arm, back
- Localized or diffuse
- Occasionally restricted to the nipple: thelalgia
- Burning sensation or a full feeling, sometimes simple pruritis
- Rhythmed or not by the cycle, pre- or sometimes postmenstrual
- Chronic or recent

Interpreting the Pain

A bilateral axillomammary fullness, especially if rhythmed by the cycle, is most likely of functional origin. Presence of an organic lesion, however, should be suspected when the pain is characterized by its type (burning, pruritis), location (unilateral, associated with a palpable abnormality), recent appearance, or persistence.

1.2.1.2 Galactorrhea

This is by definition a bilateral and multiductal lactescent discharge (which may be somewhat yellow, brown or green in color). The amount is quite variable. It may be slight and appear only after compression. Its duration and evolution as compared with the reproductive years should be noted. Galactorrhea may occur following pregnancy, with or without lactation. It may follow a period of amenorrhea or develop spontaneously.

Interpreting the Galactorrhea

Compression producing a milky droplet at the end of the menstrual cycle is not considered pathologic. Slight galactorrhea for several months after a pregnancy is also normal. It may be just one symptom of a major functional hyperactivity syndrome. In all other cases, thorough examination is essential to determine the cause of galactorrhea.

1.2.1.3 Sectorial Discharge

This type of discharge, which is unilateral, involving only one or a few ducts, is due to a localized abnormality. The amount of discharge is quite variable. It may be slight and only appear with compression. It may be possible to determine precisely the zone where the fluid originates by the "pencil sign." A pencil-like object is used to apply pressure in the direction of the ductal axes. Occasionally, the discharge is only discovered with compression during mammography. The liquid may be watery, thick, or even purulent. It may be serous, bloody (thelorrhagia), brownish, or milky. Its macroscopic appearance, however, is not an indication of its cytologic composition.

Interpreting the Sectorial Discharge

This indicates the presence of an organic abnormality: common ductal ectasia, papillary adenoma, or papillary carcinoma.

1.2.2 Physical Examination

1.2.2.1 Inspection

Technique

The seated position is preferable to the standing position (Figs. 2, 3). Good lighting is essential and best if the source can be oriented in order to view specific areas clearly. Here is an additional use for the diaphanoscope light. Changes in position: arms raised overhead or tilting the bust, may help to accentuate ceratin abnormalities.

Interpretation

From a strictly medical standpoint, there is no "norm" concerning the size and form of the breasts. Even moderate asymmetry is common. Any distinct or secondary disharmony should, however, be noted:

- Recent or considerable mammary asymmetry
- Somatomammary discordance (large breasts of a thin woman, suggesting endocrine hypertrophy or small android-type breasts of a heavy woman)

Skin and/or nipple retraction suggest an underlying tumor. This is most often benign: cyst, fibroadenoma, phylloide tumor, but sometimes malignant: malignant phylloide tumor, sarcoma, epithelioma. Congenital uni- or bilateral nipple

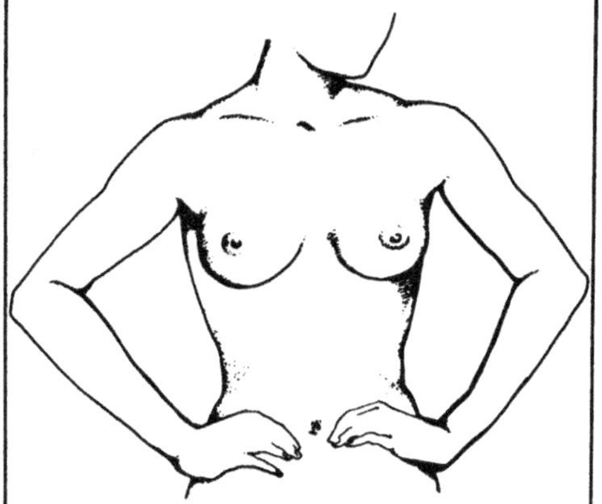

Fig. 2. Inspection

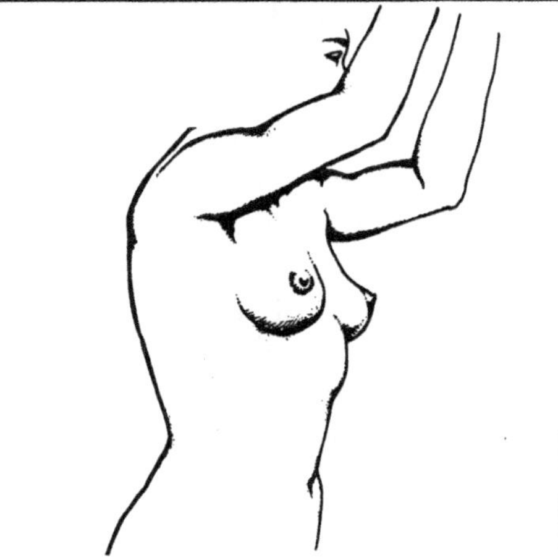

Fig. 3. Inspection

retraction would be known to the patient. Skin dimpling forming a groove is characteristic of Mondor's disease. Nipple or skin retraction is characteristic of the sclerosis that accompanies distrophy, scarring, and cancer.

Bruising indicates recent trauma. Erythema and hypervascularization are due to the different types of mastitis and inflammation. Skin and nipple changes may result from mammary disease: the small fistula of subareolar abscess, pseudoeczema of Paget's disease, ulcerated carcinoma, *"peau d'orange"* of diffuse carcinoma. Other abnormalities are specifically cutaneous. All elements on the breasts should be topographically noted since they may result in false images during mammography. For the same reason all scars should be marked on a diagram.

Strong Points

- Skin and nipple disorders: Paget's disease
- Carcinoma adherent to the skin
- Inflammatory processes

1.2.2.2 Palpation

Principle

Palpation determines the mechanical cohesion of the tissues. Both breasts as well as axillary and retroclavicular nodes are systematically examined.

Firstly, two parameters should be noted: the degree of this tissular cohesion (firm or soft breasts) and its homogeneity (homogeneous, granular, nodular breasts). Secondly, a tumor may be detected. This requires that there be a contrast in consistency between the lesion and surrounding tissue. Even if small, a hard tumor in a soft homogeneous breast will be easily detected. The same is not true when the breast is firm, heterogeneous, and large, particularly if the lesion is deep.

Technique

The examination is carried out with the patient in both sitting and supine positions. It is important to finish by examining the patient in any position where she may have felt something abnormal: bent over at the waist, elbow slightly turned, pectoral muscles slightly contracted. Equally important is the repalpation of an area found suspect by another examination technique. The breast is palpated using the flat of the last four fingers (distal extremities). Each section examined is flatenned against the ribs (Figs. 4, 5). Using measured soft and progressive pressure, the fingers make adapted rotary movements. Each nipple should be milked to determine its suppleness and mobility (Fig. 6). Each axillary region is palpated in two steps: enlarged nodes are detected first by pressing deeply against the ribs and then with the fingers hooked, against the pectoralis major (Figs. 7, 8). Supra- and subclavicular nodes are easily palpated (Fig. 9).

Interpretation

– General consistency of the breasts

Predominantly adipose breasts are generally soft but may be well supported.

Breast firmness is essentially due to hydration of the glandular stroma. Thus, the greater the amount of glandular tissue the greater degree of hydration possible. Normal consistency is homogeneous or macronodular: the fingers discern turgescent mammary lobes. Micronodular or granular consistency is characteristic of the excess hydration of distrophy.

In all cases, the ability to detect localized abnormalities depends on the breast's general consistency. The firmer the breast the less accurate the palpation.

– Well-delineated, smooth, mobile tumors

This description is characteristic of benign tumors. The consistency may help to orient the diagnosis: lipomas are soft; hamartomas are firmer; adenomas, fibroadenomas, and phylloide tumors are firmer still; cysts, encysted hematomas, abcesses, and galactoceles are liquid collections which are resistant. Some cancerous lesions, however, may have similar appearances: nodular epithelioma, colloid carcinoma, sarcoma, and intracystic carcinoma.

– Poorly delineated and/or irregular and/or fixed tumors

Each case in the preceding section may actually present with such appearances when accompanied by edema, glandular condensation or sclerosis. Simple

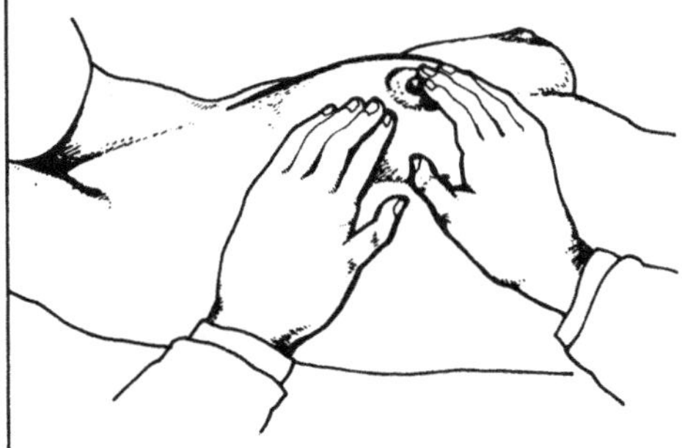

Fig. 4. Palpation in the supine position

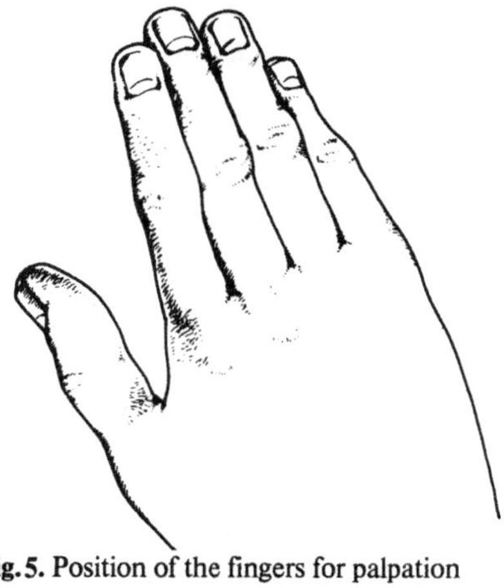

Fig. 5. Position of the fingers for palpation

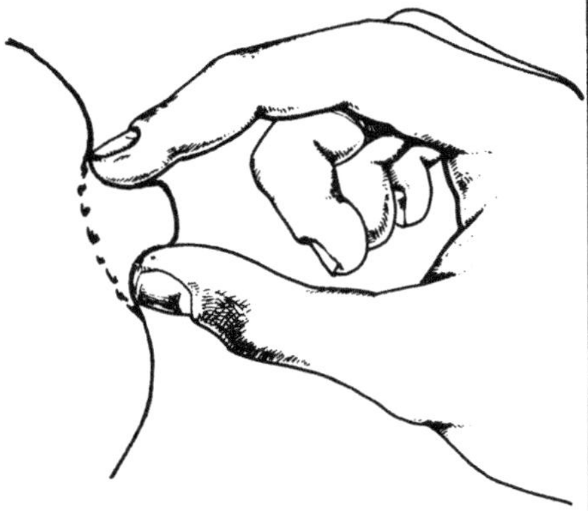

Fig. 6. Nipple palpation

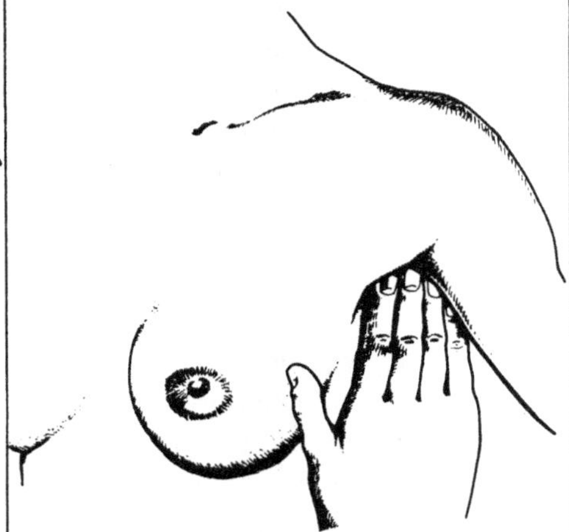

Fig. 7. Axillary palpation

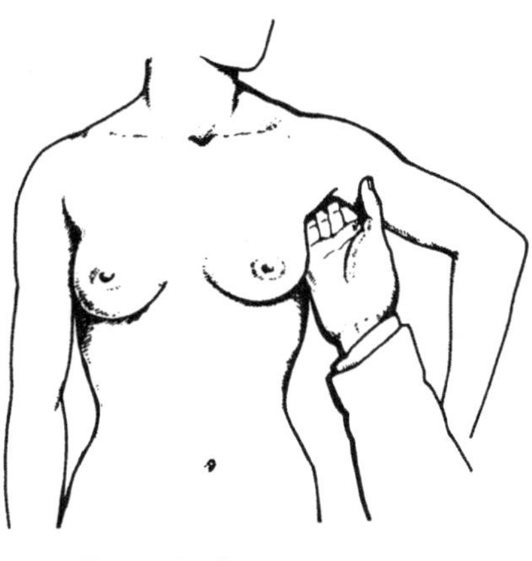

Fig. 8. Axillary palpation

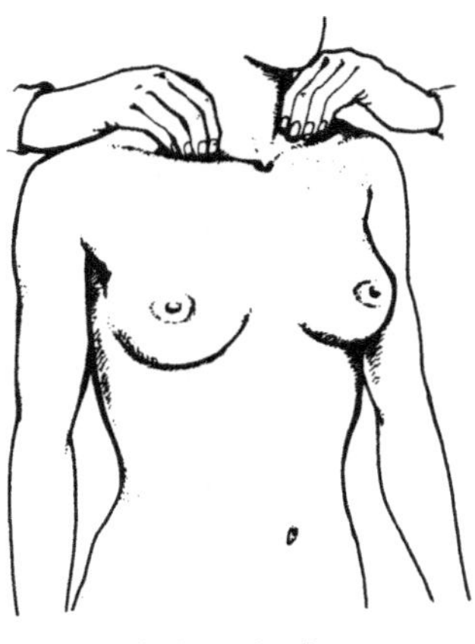

Fig. 9. Supraclavicular palpation

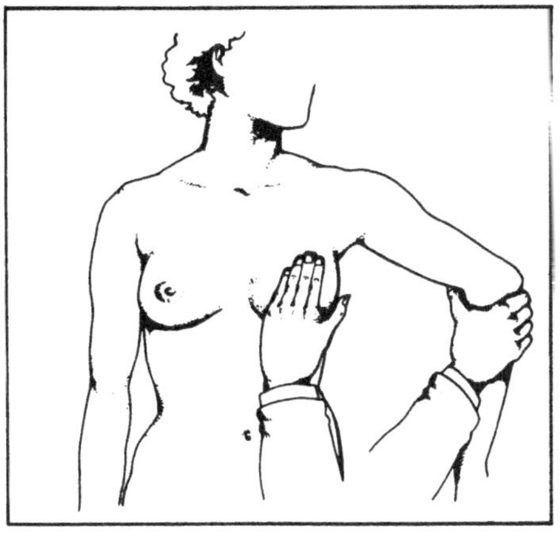

Fig. 10. Tillaux's technique

dystrophic densification without any actual anatomic lesion may also present as such, forming what we call the "nameless nodule." Despite these benign possibilities, it is cancer in all its forms, histologic types and stages that is the main consideration here.

– Describing the tumor

Once detected the following tumoral characteristics should be noted: size, site, form, consistency, and mobility. The size does not always correspond to the actual anatomic lesion. Excess pressure of the surrounding tissue cannot be distinguished from the carcinoma during palpation. Nevertheless, the palpated mass should be measured and classified according to the international classification (Table 4, p. 135). Site is determined according to one of the four quadrants of the breast. Form (as with size) is described in geometrical rather than figurative terms: round, oval, polycyclic, elongated lump or mass.

Consistency is a relative feature which depends on the surrounding tissue. It may have a particular characteristic: resistance. Pressure applied by one finger to an immobilized tumor is transmitted to another finger at a different point on the tumor. This is due to the incompressibility of fluid in a flexible but inextensible cavity. In principle, it indicates the presence of a fluid collection. Mobility of the lesion is determined by comparison with the surrounding tissue, skin, nipple, and underlying deep layers (aided by Tillaux's technique for pectoral contraction) (Fig. 10). Lymph nodes should also be described according to size, site, form, and mobility as well as classified according to the international classification (Table 4, p. 135).

1.2.2.3 Combined Palpation

Palpation is also used in conjunction with other methods of examination:

- During inspection, it helps in observing slight cutaneous or nipple retraction (Fig. 11) and *peau d'orange* due to pinching of underlying tissue (Fig. 12).

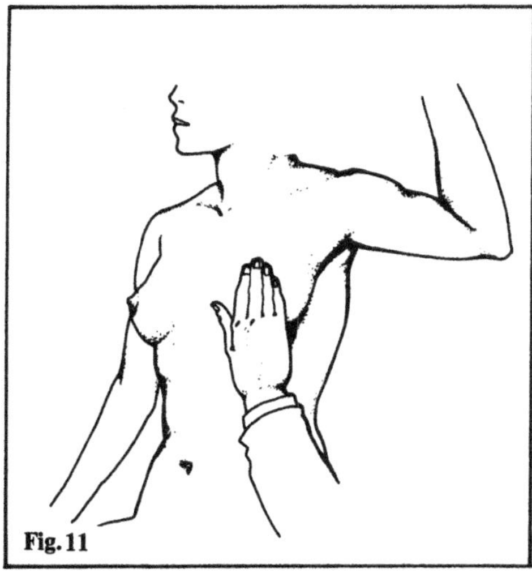

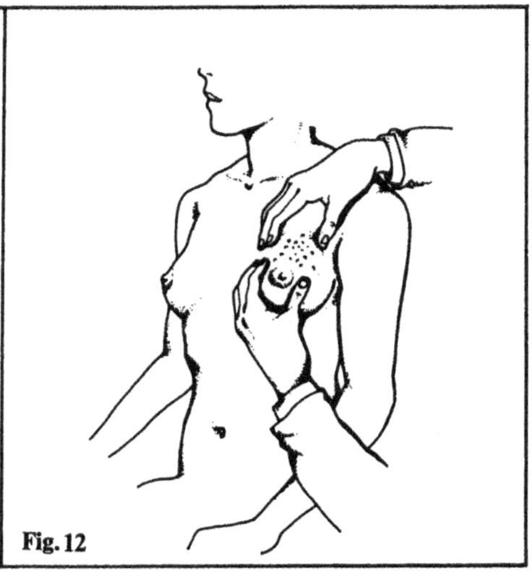

Fig. 11. Inspection/palpation: testing for skin and nipple retraction

Fig. 12. Inspection/palpation: slight compression reveals the *peau d'orange*

- During transillumination and ultrasound, it helps to locate an abnormality and determine its size.
- During mammography it helps to carry out special views: for example, a tangential view of an otherwise difficult to analyze abnormality.
- During needle aspiration it is the best method for localization.

Strong Points
- Fibroadenomas in young girls
- Postmenopausal nodular carcinoma
- Adenopathy

Weak Points
- Mastosis
- Painful lesions
- Diffuse lesions

1.3 Transillumination

Transillumination is the study of changes in a light beam passing through the breast.

1.3.1 Diaphanoscopy

1.3.1.1 Principle

In a dark room, the examiner directly observes the transilluminated breast. For an incident beam of white light, the emergent light is orange. Its intensity varies depending on the thickness and composition of the breast.

1.3.1.2 Material

Any light source can be used providing it is sufficiently powerful, cold, and small (observation is difficult if greater than 2 cm). It helps to have a wide range of light intensity.

1.3.1.3 Technique

The examination is best carried out in complete darkness. The patient sits facing the examiner. The latter holds the source against the inferior aspect of the breast

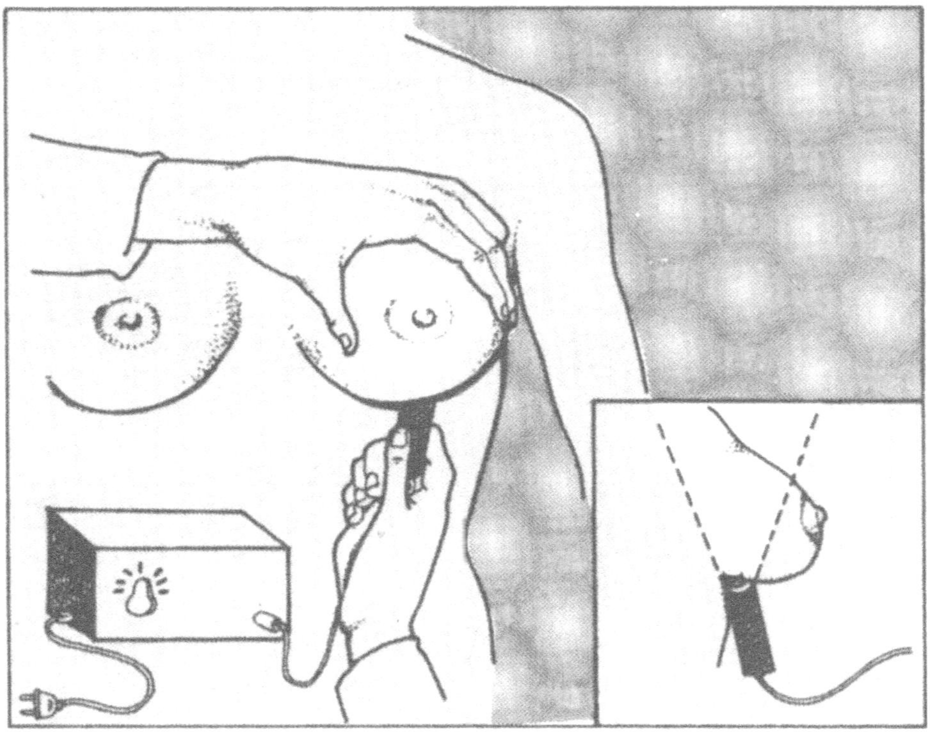

Fig. 13. Transillumination

with one hand and uses the other to move the breast in order to examine each area (Fig. 13). By varying the beam's intensity, he selects the setting which corresponds to the best contrast. It is the same principle as in fluoroscopy: if the beam is insufficient, the resulting image is inadequate; if too strong the image loses contrast due to a blinding effect.

1.3.1.4 Interpretation

General Appearances

Schematically, three images can be described:
- High homogeneous transparency corresponding to the adipose type (Fig. 14a)
- Strong overall opacity corresponding to the fibroglandular type (Fig. 14b)
- Strong contrast between the highly opaque glandular cone and the transparent subcutaneous adipose tissue corresponding to the mastosic type (Fig. 14c)

Localized Abnormalities

For a known lesion we can observe its opacity or, more precisely, the contrast between this opacity and that of the surrounding tissue:
- High transparency suggests a lipoma or clear fluid cyst (Fig. 15a)

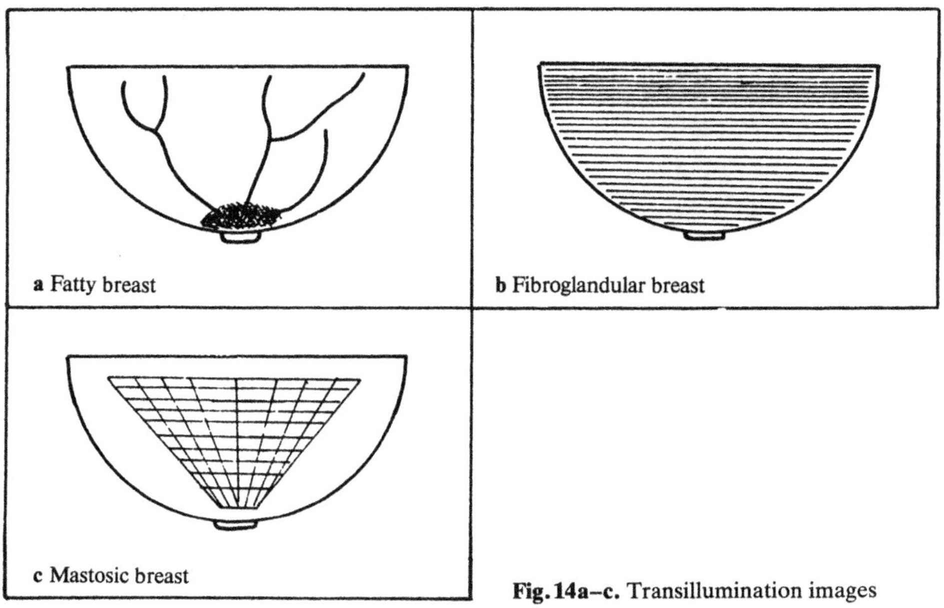

Fig. 14a–c. Transillumination images

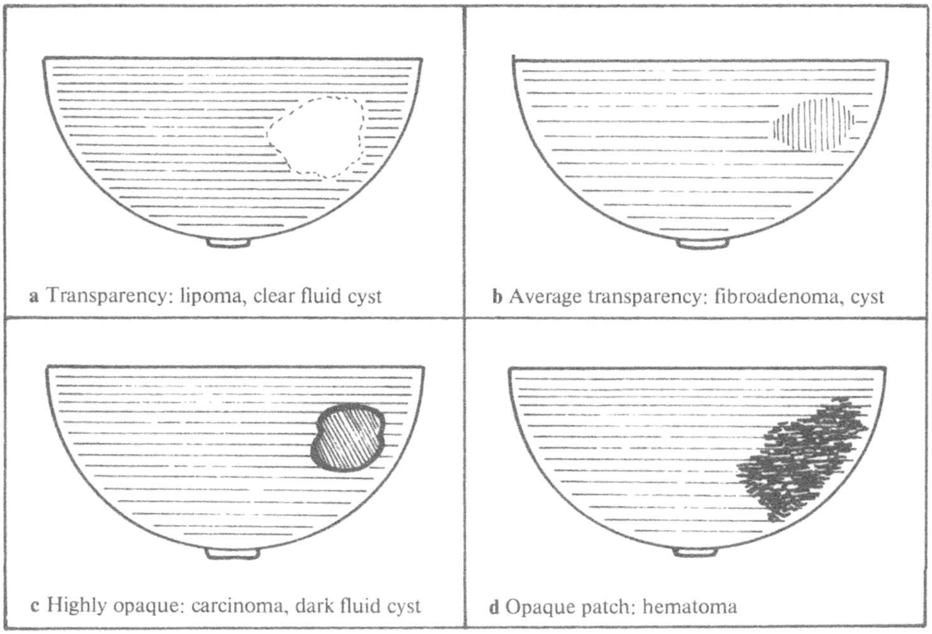

Fig. 15a–d. Localized transillumination abnormalities

- Average transparency is characteristic of mastosic nodules, fibroadenomas, and cysts (Fig. 15b)
- Strong opacity suggests carcinoma or dark fluid cysts (Fig. 15c)

When a lesion has not previously been detected, transillumination may demonstrate a distinct opacity. A good example is the hematoma (Fig. 15d), which often goes undetected by other examination techniques. Occasionally a small distinct opacity is discovered in an area where other examinations failed to demonstrate an abnormality. Since it is not well understood, this sign should be taken into consideration according to each particular case. It is important to underline the relativity of the images. As in mammography, transillumination uses the changes in a beam of electromagnetic radiation through the breast. It only shows contrast, and resolution is too weak to create the "edge effect" observed in radiology. In addition, with the diffusion phenomenon being predominant here, the thickness of the lesion compared with that of the breast plays an even more important role than in mammography for the formation of an image.

Strong Points
- Hematoma
- Suspicious zone in diffuse distrophy

Weak Point
- Small lesion in an opaque breast

1.3.2 Diaphanometry

1.3.2.1 Principle

Transparency of the breast to a light beam depends on its thickness and the cellular density of the tissue. For a given thickness, the measure of the emergent light intensity constitutes a parameter indicative of the type of tissue (the incident light intensity being constant). Two findings, therefore, should be simultaneously obtained: the thickness traversed and the emergent light intensity.

1.3.2.2 Material

The equipment used today will probably be improved upon in the future. Here, we describe that which we feel to be the best at the moment.
- Light source: 0–300 W, cooled lamp
- Transmission of light to the breast: by a bundle of glass fibers
- Recording apparatus: two adjustable electronically measured parallel plates; a photoelectric cell on one of the plates facing the end of the glass fiber bundle attached to the other plate; and an electronic recording device connected to the cell

1.3.2.3 Technique

The examination is carried out under the same conditions as transillumination. The breast is placed between the two plates, which are moderately tightened. By varying the rheostat of the light beam's supply circuit, the emergent beam is adjusted to the required setting. The diaphanometric index is read directly on the control dial of the rheostat (Fig. 16). Physically, the resulting figure only has a relative value but is significant of the type of tissue for a given thickness. Many measurements would still be necessary to establish a law of thickness which could make use of a single value scale.

1.3.2.4 Interpretation

Attenuation of the beam depends primarily on the number of microscopic scale elements. Strong absorption is characteristic of mastosis with epithelial prolifer-

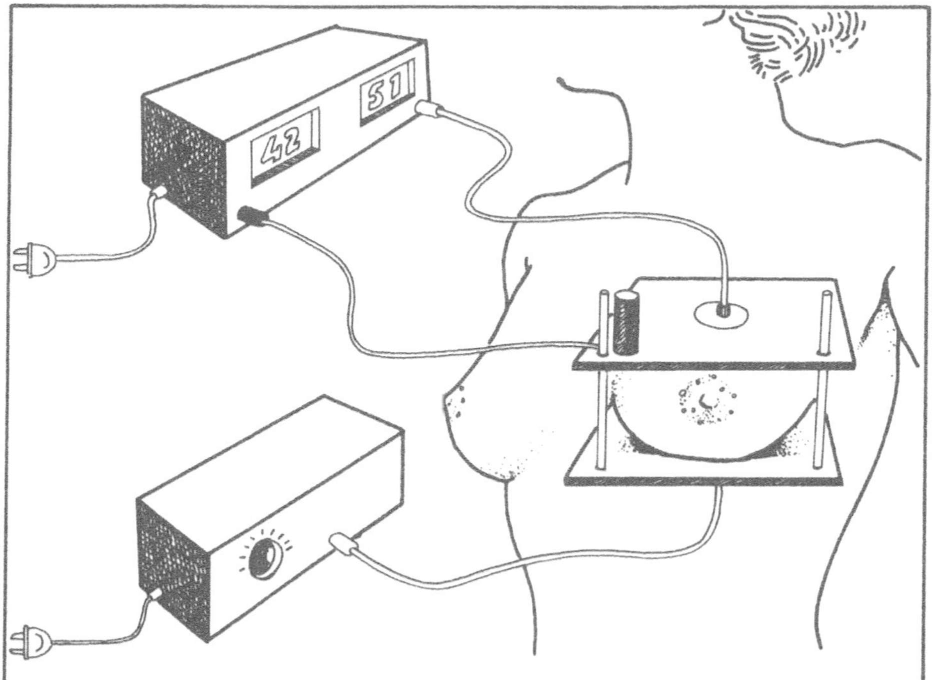

Fig. 16. Diaphanometry

ation; weak absorption is due to predominantly adipose tissue; excess hydration of glandular stroma promotes passage of the light beam (while increasing the thickness of the breast).

Strong Point
Diagnosis of mastosis or, more particularly, differential diagnosis between mastosis (opaque) and functional excess hydration of the stroma (translucent)

Weak Point
Still in the research stage

1.3.2.5 Somanetics

According to studies by R. L. Egan, Atlanta (unpublished) the Somanetics Corporation of Troy, Michigan has developed computer associated diaphanometry. A series of measurements are made at four points in each breast. ... This method shows promise but requires further research.

1.4 Ultrasonography

Through its different forms ultrasonography studies changes in a beam of ultrasound vibrations penetrating the breast. The information it provides is related to the physical composition of breast tissues.

1.4.1 A Mode

1.4.1.1 Principle

The transmitter-receiver transducer emits an ultrasound beam along an axis. On emission, the signals are short and discontinuous. At reentry, the transducer receives reflected waves along the same axis. The reentry time is used to establish the distance between the transducer and the point of the echo's emission. A curve is thus produced on an oscilloscope with the echo's depth along the abscissa and its intensity along the ordinate. Each echo is due to an interface or passage from one medium to another of different acoustic impedance. Dense tissue contains many interfaces and in principle creates numerous echoes. The unit, however, only records those signals returning along its exploration axis. Other echoes are lost. Highly unstructured tissue, such as carcinoma, creates few echoes and at the same time greatly attenuates the beam.

1.4.1.2 Material

The transducer contains a piezoelectric element, which is placed in contact with the skin. It is linked by a cable to a high-frequency current generator and echo signal receptor. Depending on the unit, frequencies used for the breast vary between 3.5 and 7 mHz (1 mHz = 1 million vibrations per second). The higher the frequency, the better the lateral resolution, but penetration decreases. The curve is observed directly on the oscilloscope. It may be recorded on ECG-type paper or by screen photography. The gain adjustment control is graduated, making it possible to calculate the attenuation or reinforcement effect of a lesion on the beam's intensity.

1.4.1.3 Technique

The patient is seated, inclined, or supine. A ultrasonography is used for a palpated lesion. The lesion is immobilized with one hand while the other hand places the transducer perpendicular to the skin, which is pretreated with an oil or gel contact substance. The observed (and eventually recorded) curve shows the lesion's depth, size, echogenic behavior, and effect on the beam's intensity. The gain is then adjusted in order to bring the echoes produced by the lesion up to their "normal" value. This difference, expressed in decibels, corresponds to the degree of the attenuation or reinforcement effect of the lesion.

1.4.1.4 Interpretation

We can establish a simplified classification:

- Adipose tissue contains few cellular elements and thus produces few echoes. It only slightly weakens the beam.
- Normal lactiferous connective tissue moderately reflects and absorbs and thus in each case serves as a reference for calibrating the gain which the sonographer does for each case (Fig. 17a).
- Cystic contents, the ideal homogeneous medium, are sonolucent. They are not only homogeneous, but in no way attenuate the beam. By comparison with the surrounding tissue, we observe a relative reinforcement of the intensity of the beam, and thus the echoes, after passage through the cyst (a progressive echo reinforcement device is used to compensate the inevitable energy loss with penetration. This explains why echoes may appear more intense once through a cyst than before) (Fig. 17b).

  That the form of the cyst can be modified by external changes in pressure is also demonstrated by this technique.
- A solid benign lesion sometimes produces more echoes but often fewer than normal tissue. It does not, however, increase beam attenuation (Fig. 17c).
- Carcinoma is hypoechogenic and hyperabsorbant (Fig. 17d). It does not change shape: by applying pressure to the lesion with the transducer, the image of the lesion moves without changing form. Attenuation of the beam by the lesion can be calculated.

In practice, it suffices to refer to the basic trends in the above list:

- Slightly modified beam: dystrophic lesion
- Reinforced beam: fluid collection
- Highly attenuated beam: carcinoma

Not only can all intermediates be observed, but this basic outline is of little use when a lesion has particular mechanical properties due to its structure:

- A cyst may emit echoes and weaken the beam if it contains thick or pasty fluid
- A benign solid lesion may have sclerous areas with an absorption pattern similar to that of carcinoma
- Some forms of carcinoma (colloid, comedocarcinoma) which are relatively homogeneous may simulate benign forms in A ultrasound.

It is interesting to observe how the curve is modified when additional pressure is applied to the transducer: a cyst changes shape: its diameter decreases while a solid lesion moves without change in diameter.

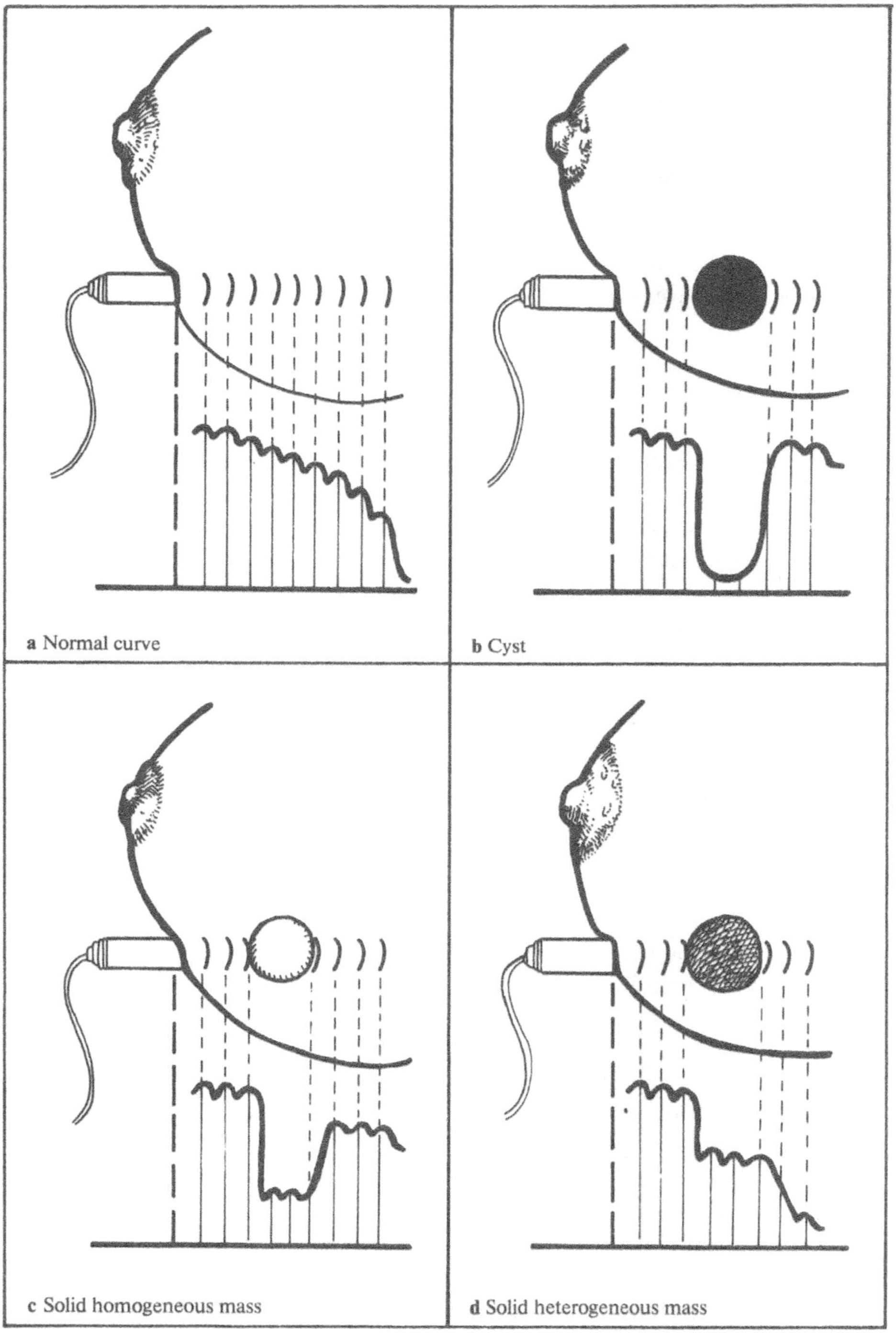

a Normal curve

b Cyst

c Solid homogeneous mass

d Solid heterogeneous mass

Fig. 17a–d. A mode ultrasonography: results

A ultrasound may be used for guided puncture. When the lesion is viewed on the screen its depth and size, as well as the direction of the transducer, is noted. These findings help to place the needle correctly. Use of an adapted transducer through which the needle can be passed makes it possible to puncture without interrupting the curve.

Strong Point
Study of a previously detected lesion

Weak Point
As a screening technique

1.4.2 B Mode (Echotomography)

1.4.2.1 Principle

It is the same as in A mode except that, instead of a single axis, a two-dimensional area is explored which produces an image: this is echotomography. In A ultrasound, the axis was represented by a curve. Here it is represented by a line, each point of which is either light or dark depending on whether or not it represents an echo. Echoes may show black on a white background; however, the reverse is generally preferred since it is more comfortable for the eye. Much more extensive information is provided by the spectrum of grays instead of all or nothing: echo or no echo, implying the existence of a threshold. The instrument records slight variations of gray corresponding to the echo intensity at each point. By moving the transducer or, with a series of aligned transducers (multiple linear array transducers), a tomographic image is produced: a juxtaposition of the lines forming the explored section.

1.4.2.2 Material

Diverse methods of applying this basic principle are technically possible and the choice for the breast is an area of controversy. We will defend our present choice, point by point, based on daily use of the technique, as well as indicate the actual performance of each type of equipment.

Manual or Automatic Scanning?

In the former case, the sonologist uses a small transducer identical to the A-mode type. The image of each line is electronically frozen on the screen, thus creating a stable tomographic image. In the latter case, scanning is slow (static image) or rapid (dynamic or "real time" image).

Manual scanning produces the best quality image. Technical restrictions of automatic scanning give poorer quality results. While highly efficient for examining a palpated lesion, the manual method is not adapted to the indispensable detection examination which explores the entire organ, whether or not a palpable lesion is present. In addition, the mobility of some breasts make scanning of a given lesion particularly tedious. Automatic scanning, therefore, is our choice.

Slow Automatic Scanning[1] *or Real Time?*

It makes sense to consider slow scanning, which has the best resolution. The image is formed by means of one or several transducers moved with precision along the examined section.

The entire device is moved in order to examine different areas of the breast. Resulting images are particularly interesting since they show the form of the breast as well as the chest wall. Resolution is fairly good. This technique does have serious drawbacks in addition to being cumbersome and its cost. For screening purposes the complete examination is long, approximately ¼ h. It inconveniently isolates the patient from the physician since she must be in the prone position with her breasts in a fluid-filled pocket. Its major disadvantage is the impossibility of using the essential combination palpation-ultrasound.

For these reasons, we prefer real time scanning.

Electronic or Mechanical Real Time?

In the former case, the transducer is composed of a series of crystals in linear array. Each element is successively activated. A complete image can be observed since the process is repetitive and the scanning time short: inferior to the total retentivity of the screen and eye. All lines forming the image are parallel.

In the latter case, one transducer (sometimes three), once activated, functions constantly. It moves rapidly within a casing containing transmission fluid. The image is sectorial since the axes explored diverge to a certain degree. The moving axis, however, may be sufficiently distant so that the line of contact is fairly long (at least 6 cm).

Due to undeniable physical laws, the first centimeter of tissue cannot be studied. In breast examination this first centimeter is particularly important. Thus, the major advantage of mechanical scanning in breast examination is that it functions in a fluid pocket so that the crystal is removed from the skin.

It is possible to use a linear array and interpose a small water bag. We have run a few trials which appear promising but not to the point of discontinuing mechanical scanning.

---

1 Mistakenly referred to as "scanner"

What Type of Mechanical Scanning?

We use simple equipment, whose basic features have proven satisfactory. Major improvements are still necessary but have not as yet been provided by the engineer. In other words, what we will describe here is an ideal unit.

The sectorial scanner should be easy to handle and as light as possible. Otherwise, it should rest on a movable support so that the sonologist does not have to concentrate all his effort on holding the transducer.

In order clearly to identify the examined area, contact with the skin should be as close as possible. Physical characteristics of the transducer should provide the best resolution compatible with the necessary penetration. The frequency should be at least 5 mHz with good beam focalization.

The parameters of the curve should be easy to see and adjust. It is possible to reproduce the image, once frozen, without any notable loss of detail (on X-ray film or paper). It helps to have calipers: an instrument used for measuring the distance between two points on the screen.

It should be possible to obtain an A echo with a monodirectional transducer. At the same time the echotomographic image appears on the screen, it is particularly interesting to project the A curve corresponding to an axis seen on the B image.

Under the same conditions, the TM mode (see p. 27) can be a valuable aid.

1.4.2.3 Technique

The patient is in the supine position. Contact substance is abundantly applied. One hand holds the transducer perpendicular to the skin; the other guides while palpating, with the nipple used as a reference point, and makes the necessary adjustments on the control panel. For each breast, cutaneous and subcutaneous layers as well as the deepest glandular tissue should be simultaneously observed. Whether or not a lesion is detected, both breasts should be completely examined. At least one film should be taken of a lesion.

1.4.2.4 Interpretation

Anatomical Features (Fig. 18)

- Skin is seen as an echogenic band several millimeters thick.
- Subcutaneous adipous tissue in which the mammary crests are found is very weakly echogenic.
- Glandular tissue varies in density according to the type of structure.
- Retromammary fatty tissue is sonolucent.

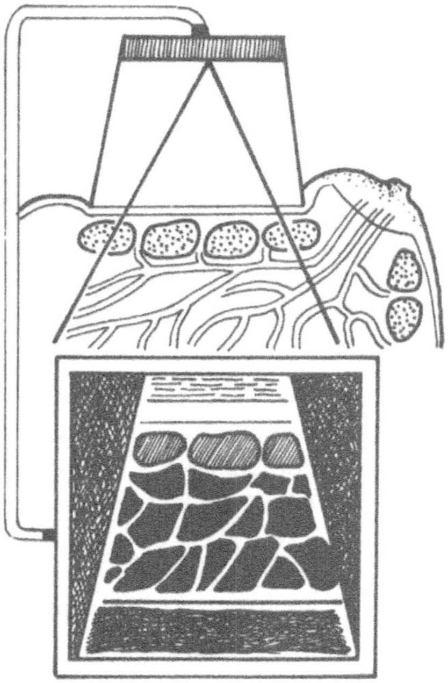

Fig. 18. Normal tissue

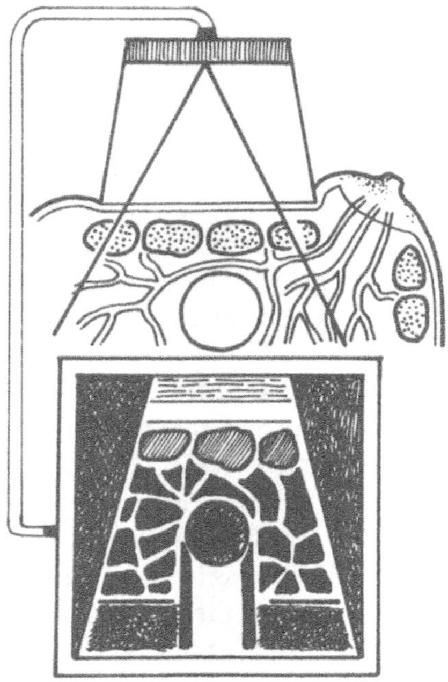

Fig. 19. Fluid cavity

Figs. 18, 19. B mode ultrasonography: results

- The ribs are represented by a series of regularly aligned, clearly delineated lacunae.

Type of Tissue

Echogenic characteristics of the different tissues provide distinctive sonographic images:

- Glandular tissue is highly echogenic. A breast with epithelial proliferation or simply a high percentage of glandular tissue will have a very white image (white mode on black).
- Adipous tissue is weakly echogenic. A breast lacking in glandular tissue has a dark image (predominantly black) in which connective tissue provides strong contrast.
- Hydration makes tissues more sonolucent. This occurs primarily in the perilobular spaces, creating a schematic appearance on the sonogram by accentuating interlobular outlines. Full alveoli will scatter the image with microlacunae.

Localized Lesions

These are defined by: site, size, form, outline, type (hypo- or hyperechogenic), structure (homogeneous or not), and their effect on the beam's intensity: reinforcement, absorption, lateral shadows.

Site

Measuring devices usually integrated into the unit will easily determine depth. The exact topography must be carefully established, taking into consideration the patient's supine position, the position of the arms, and the effect of the transducer on the breast's position.

Size and Form

These are determined according to two directions perpendicular to each other. Images correspond to the lesion's external contour. A certain discordance may arise with a cyst since the contour demonstrated by cystography corresponds to the inner cavity.

Outline

Ultrasound will determine how well it is delineated. It is important to consider the physical conditions involved in the formation of the outline.

- Anterior contours may be blurred by repeated echoes.
- Lateral outlines may partially blend into lateral shadows.
- Posterior outlines form according to changes in the beam having passed through the lesion: they are underlined in a cyst and effaced in carcinoma.

Sonographic Type

Isoechogenic Formation

A lesion may go undectected if it has the same echogenicity as surrounding tissues. Occasionally a questionable outline will appear. This is particularly the case with nodular dystrophic lesions in mastosis and with hamartomas.

Hypoechogenic Formation

A perfect example is the lacuna, the most frequent pathologic sonographic image.

- A lacuna with no echoes corresponds to a homogeneous medium without interfaces such as a fluid collection. A cyst with its regular and rounded wall

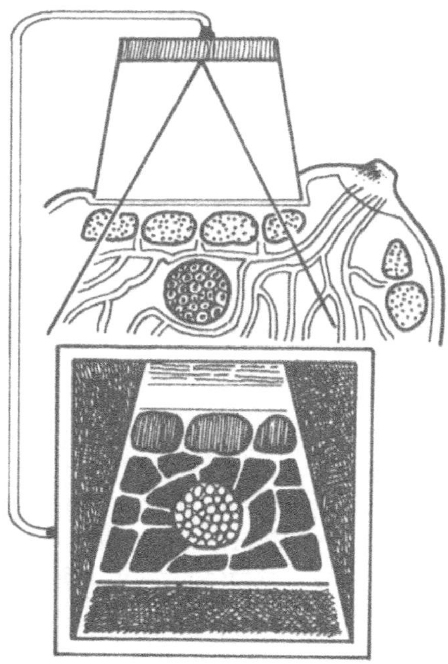

Fig. 20. Solid homogeneous mass (benign type)

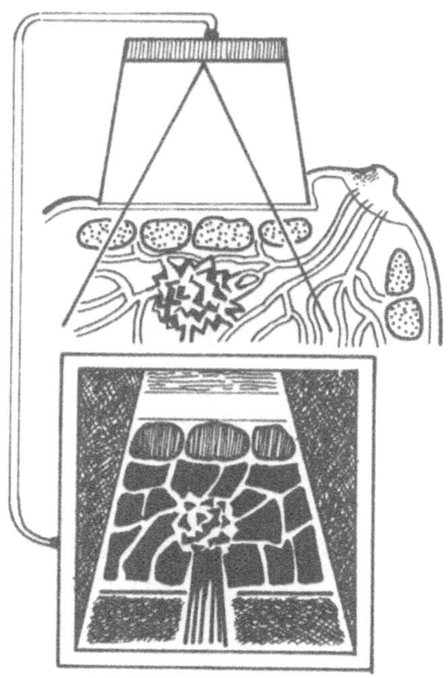

Fig. 21. Solid heterogeneous mass (malignant type)

has a characteristic appearance: the tangent effect causes blurring of the lateral contours and the formation of shadow lines; integral transmission of the beam underlines the posterior contour of the lacuna and reinforces the beam's intensity behind the lesion (Fig. 19).

- A lacuna with evenly distributed echoes suggests the homogeneous structure of a benign lesion: rare echoes of a lipoma, islets of denser echoes of a hamartoma, fairly intense echoes of adenomas, fibroadenomas, and phylloide tumors. These lesions do not attenuate and may even reinforce the beam. They form lateral shadows if their outlines are regular (Fig. 20).
- A lacuna with irregularly distributed echoes suggests the anarchic structure of carcinoma (Fig. 21).

This simplified classification has the same nuances as that of ultrasound A (cf. p. 21).

Strong Points

- Highly dense breasts
- Cysts
- Benign lesions

Weak Points
- Adipose breasts
- Small and/or deep lesions

1.4.3 TM Mode (Time Motion)

1.4.3.1 Principle

This is the recording of variations of an A sonogram over time. Consider the A curve on the screen, not as a curve, but as a line of points varying in intensity as in B ultrasound. Like the tracing of a graph, variations of this line can be recorded by appearing and remaining on the screen at fairly close intervals of time.

This method is especially valuable for moving organs, particularly the heart.

The TM mode is also useful for studying the behavior of a tumor in a solid organ by varying the pressure applied to the transducer.

1.4.3.2 Material

This is an electrical unit joined to an A or B ultrasound unit. The visual screen may be part of, or separate from, the other modes. The image is produced at different speeds and is referenced with respect to time. The image can be frozen and photographed.

1.4.3.3 Technique

The A mode is used to position correctly the transducer over the lesion. For some B mode units, TM is produced according to an axis chosen by the sonologist.

Strong Point
Detection of peritumoral infiltration

1.4.3.4 Interpretation

Under pressure exerted by the transducer, cysts will change shape while solid masses move without changing from (Fig. 22). TM clearly demonstrates the overall movement of adjacent areas in the case of peritumoral, especially malignant, infiltration (Fig. 23).

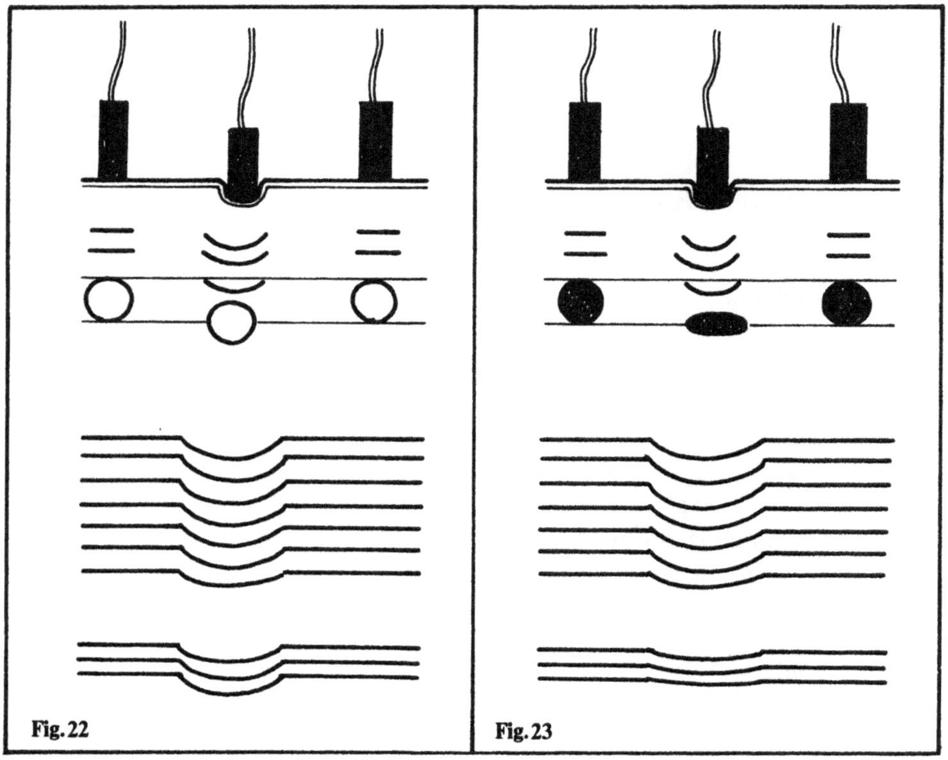

Fig. 22. Ultrasonography: TM mode. Movement without mass distortion: solid mass. Movement without distortion of surrounding tissues: infiltration

Fig. 23. Ultrasonography: TM mode. Flexible tumor: cyst

1.4.4 C Mode

This technique is still in the experimental stage but is sure to play an important role in breast examination. It creates a two-dimensional image of which each point is equidistant from the skin. The result is a transverse section as in radiology. Hopefully, the C mode will provide an important complement to clinical findings and especially to mammography, as breast positioning can be identical in both.

1.4.5 Transsonography

This is the study of changes in an ultrasound beam having passed through the breast. While still experimental, like CT, it uses a computer to record slight changes in speed used to establish the nature of the different tissues. While a distinct hope for the future, transsonography is not yet likely to modify current breast examination procedure.

1.5 Roentgenographic Diagnosis

Here, we consider the diagnostic techniques using X-rays without artificial contrast: mammography; and with artificial contrast: galactography and cystography. We conclude this section with a discussion of tomographic procedures.

1.5.1 Mammography

1.5.1.1 Principle

The radiologic image is produced by modifications of the X-ray beam within the breast. Photons of two origins reach the film: those of primary radiation, varying in number at each point depending on the obstacles encountered, which produces the useful image; and those of secondary radiation emitted by the largest obstacles. These are interference rays which are diffuse and indistinguishable from primary rays. There may be so much that it blurs the image. The breast is an organ particularly refractory to radiographic examination. Not only is its anatomic position variable but its different tissues all absorb X-rays in a similar manner. A radiologic examination should represent the best compromise between maximum quality of the image (resolution and contrast) and the least amount of radiation. The best performance can only be achieved through a constant critical and objective evaluation of the technique in question. In the same way that a chain is only as strong as its weakest link, a radiologic image owes its quality to the least efficient step in its formation. It is important to remember that contrast and resolution are related and thus it is impossible to improve one while neglecting the other (xerography, discussed later, is a special case with regard to this problem).

This technical adjustment must be made case by case since differences from one patient to another are considerable; even greater, for example, than between a wrist and a cranium. Between roentgenographs of the latter two, the radiologist not only changes constants, but also the technique (film, screens, grids). The same is true for mammography.

How a radiologic image is formed should always be present in the reader's mind:

The Radiologic Image is Composed of Contrast and Outlines

Contrasts are the result of differences in X-ray absorption within the organ. The absorption itself is related to the atomic mass of the tissue's components and its thickness.

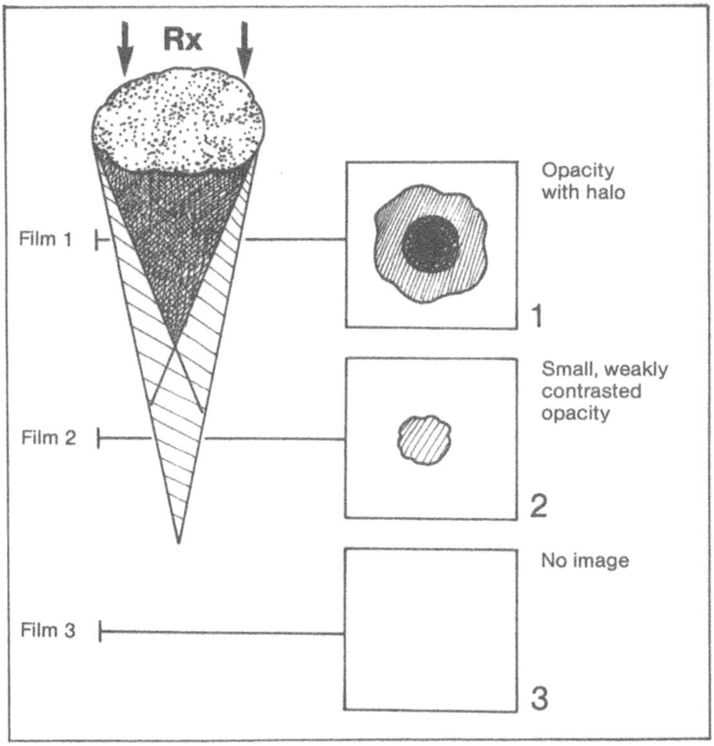

Fig. 24. Factors affecting the perception of radiographic details: *a)* Apparent size of the focal spot. Depends on the actual size of the spot and the distances: focal spot – object and focal spot – film (enlargement coefficient = FF/FO). *b)* Secondary radiation. It affects the size and contrast of the image depending on the distance: object – film (diagram). *c)* Resolution of the film or film-screen

Contours here are related to the geometric form of the tissue. They are actually the result of the beam's intensity gradient. If the intensity change occurs over a long distance, the outline is blurred. At most, it disappears and slight differences in opacity become difficult to distinguish (Fig. 24). Conversely, the shorter the distance, the more distinct the image. At the extreme, an "edge effect" can be observed which tends to "schematize" the image. This occurs in radiology and is even more pronounced in xerography. This geometric effect of the outline is all the more significant as it forms images to which the human eye is sensitive, whereas quantitative differences in tonality are only discerned after a certain threshold. This explains why, under certain circumstances, a 2-mm vessel is more easily seen than a poorly deliniated 2-cm tumor.

The Radiographic Image is Additive

Except for elements seen tangentially and for tomography, tissues are always superimposed. Always remember that the breast is a three-dimensional organ.

It is only too easy for the radiologist to imagine the breast as a triangle as represented by mammograhy when it is in fact a volume whose elements cast shadows. What is seen as the cutaneous outline represents only a small band of skin tangentially touched by the beam. The same is true for subcutaneous fatty tissue and Cooper's ligaments: subcutaneous fatty tissue transparency as well as skin and ligament opacities are spread throughout the mammographic image.

1.5.1.2 Material

An attractive exterior is not to be discarded but is not a test of the unit's quality either.

X-Ray Generator

The X-ray generator should be as powerful as possible in order to reduce the exposure time. This is not so much due to the kinetic blur, as the breast is easily immobilized, but especially for the patient's comfort. Theoretically, triphase is better than monophase since it should achieve maximum power at the desired voltage. In practice, this advantage of triphase is not as evident. A molybdenum anode should lower the high voltage to 25 kV and a tungsten anode to 20 kV.

X-Ray Tube

It is best that this tube be used exclusively for mammography. Other roentgenographic examinations, even for small bones, require a higher voltage of at least 50 kV. This may cause slight metal buildup on the tube's window, causing filtration which is acceptable in conventional radiology but strongly interferes at lower voltages.

Ordinary tungsten anodes can be used. They do, however, require a very low voltage and thus a relatively high level of radiation. Molybdenum anodes are preferable since this metal has a characteristic emission spectrum with a voltage of 27 kV appropriate for mammography (Fig. 25). This assures high efficiency and reduces the harmful and unnecessary irradiation of low-energy rays which do not reach the film. The ideal size of the focal spot depends on the distance focal spot-film. For a distance of 60 cm, good results are obtained with a 0.6-cm focal spot. The direct enlargement technique, used by some, requires a small focal spot of no more than 0.3 cm. The smaller the focal spot, the lower the

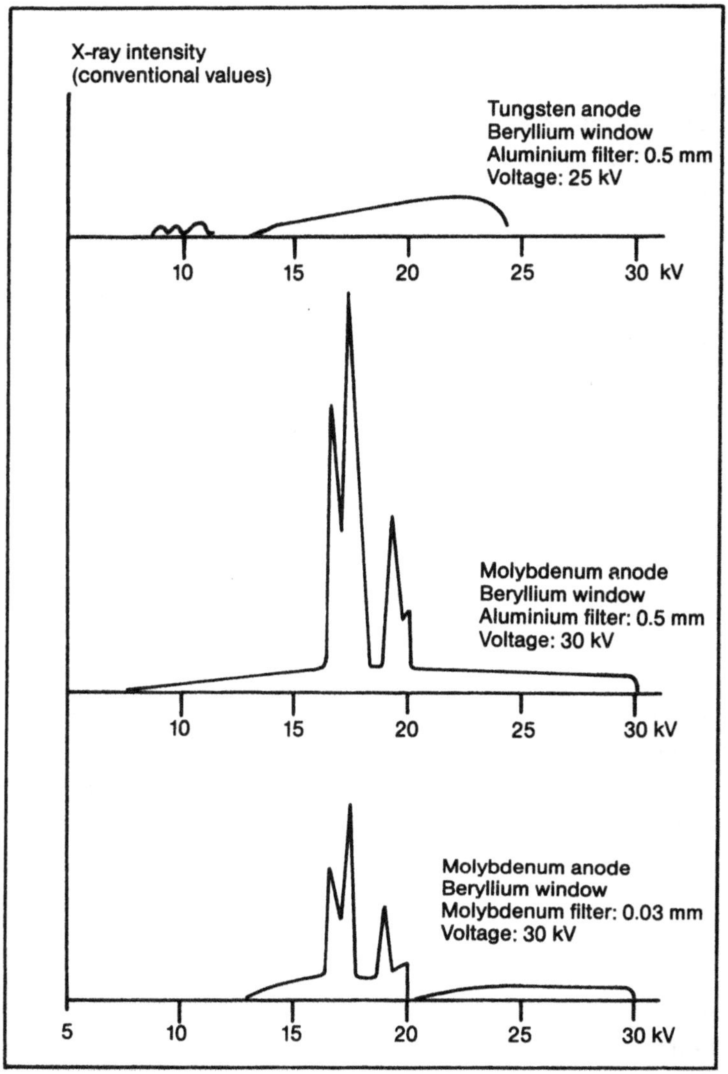

Fig. 25. Emission spectrum depending on the type of anode and the filtration

tube's power. This can be improved with the electron canon which can supply enough power with a focal spot of 0.1 cm.

In special mammography tubes, the window is composed of beryllium, which reduces absorption.

The filter at the end of the tube should be interchangeable: either 0.5 mm of aluminum providing protective filtration, or 0.3 mm of molybdenum providing specific filtration which is permeable to rays in the desired range but, on the whole, absorbs much more than aluminum.

Excellent results can be obtained without filtration but this practice must be prohibited due to the danger of very low energy rays.

The Collination Cone

This plays a double role in reducing the X-ray beam to required dimensions.
- By reducing irradiation to the patient and personnel
- By lowering secondary irradiation which distorts the image

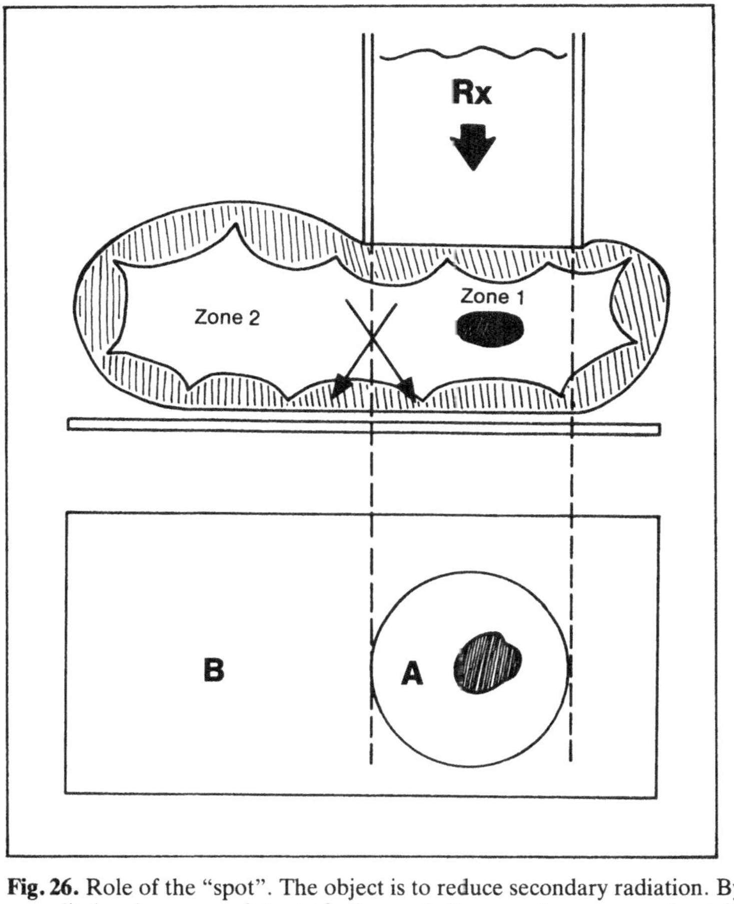

Fig. 26. Role of the "spot". The object is to reduce secondary radiation. By eliminating primary radiation from zone 2 *(outside the spot),* its secondary rays are kept from interfering with that part of the film to be studied (area *A*). Secondary rays from zone 1 *(examined),* however, will reach area *B* of the film. Actually, the resulting halo measures no more than 1 mm. In other words, the effect of the spot on secondary radiation is negligible. There are, however, some cases where local compression by the "spot" is considered to be effective. The best solution would be localized compression without the cone. For the breast, which is relatively soft, this would improve the image by decreasing thickness without obstructing localization of both lesion and image as is the case with small cones

Different types of collination devices can be used. The most efficient are flat on the side facing the patient. Others may be polyhedral or rounded. Size is of little importance. It is sometimes tempting to improve the radiologic study of a lesion by using a small "spot" collination cone. Results are more often unimpressive and it is rare that localized compression significantly improves image quality compared with good overall compression. The effect on secondary irradiation in the breast, as opposed to thick and dense organs, is negligible. In order to convince you that use of the spot in mammography is unnecessary, note how sharp the film appears: no secondary irradiation from the irradiated zone reaches outside the circle. This proves that, without the cone, secondary irradiation from outside the circle would not have struck within it (Fig. 26).

The Stand

This stabilizes the gain containing the tube. The cone, compression device, and film holder are attached to the stand. The entire unit should turn so the beam can be directed horizontally or vertically. In most cases, the examination is performed with the patient seated. The standing position is rarely used. The only logical use of the supine position is for the oblique view (lateral profile) in xerographpy, which does not require supported compression.

It makes sense that compression does not modify the distance between tube and film. In other words, compression caused by moving the tube-collination cone should be avoided. In addition, this makes it difficult to view the breast, easily verify its position, and remove wrinkles in the skin. Thus, compression should be done between two plates as gradually as possible but with sufficient force. Pneumatic systems are effective for this purpose.

The Automatic Exposure Device

This may offer satisfactory results in the hands of experts, who are often sufficiently trained so that the device is unnecessary.

The Grid

When total breast opacity increases significantly, image quality is impaired for two reasons, which are often combined:

- Either water strongly impregnates the tissues giving them an almost homogeneous density which interferes with X-ray discrimination
- Or secondary irradiation emitted by heavy tissues severely blurs the constrasts

In conventional radiology, the grid has proven effective against secondary rays. It made sense, then, to use it in mammography.

A first attempt was made with the "slit" unit. The X-ray beam is restricted by two pairs of opaque plates placed between the tube and the breast and separated by a narrow slit. Another set of plates is placed between the breast and the film. The three pairs of plates are joined together and the unit absorbs a major part of the secondary irradiation. In order to produce a complete image, the unit is moved aside (Fig. 27).

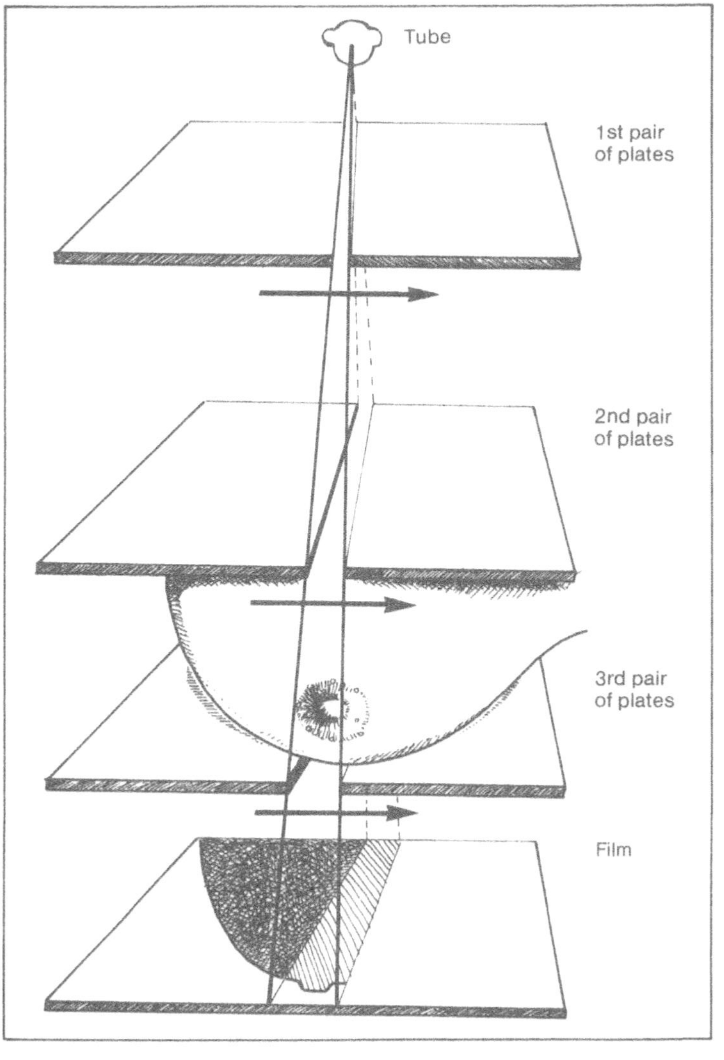

Fig. 27. Principle of the slit grid unit

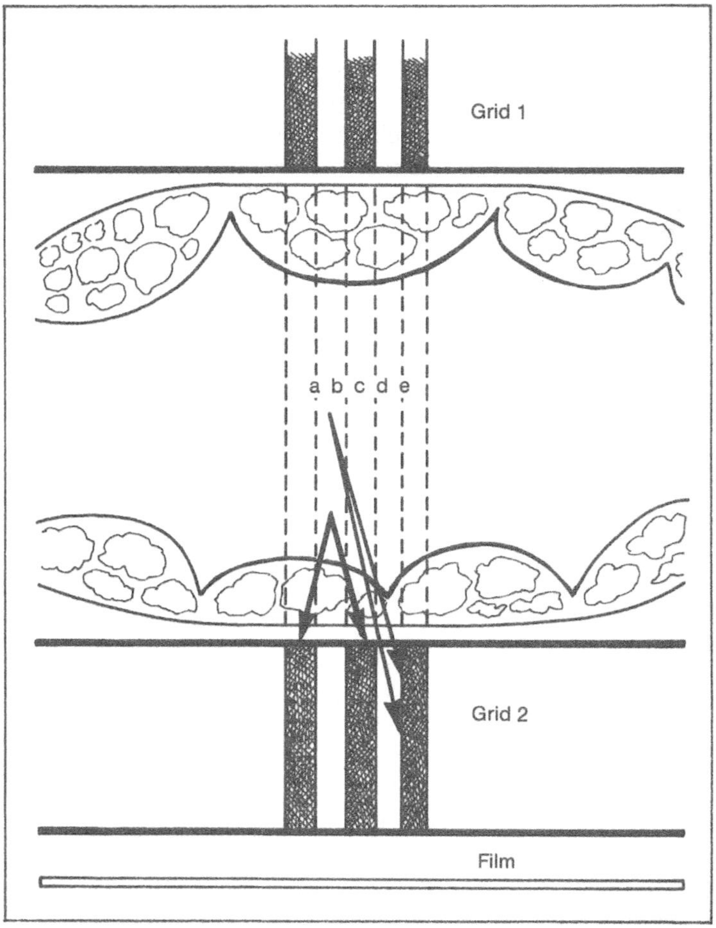

Fig. 28. Principle of the double grid. Grid 2 absorbs secondary rays whose direction differs from that of primary rays. Grid 1 protects the breast from unnecessary primary radiation corresponding to bands a, c, e, etc. At the same time, it eliminates any secondary radiation that would have resulted from these unnecessary primary rays

This system undeniably improves images of highly opaque breasts. A disadvantage is the need for strong and prolonged radiation. The patient is protected but the anode tube is overworked.

Classically designed grids are presently being used. Made of thin lead plates, separated by aluminum sheets, they represent an advantage over the slit unit in that shorter exposure times are possible. While the grid absorbs some of the secondary rays, it also absorbs part of the direct radiation otherwise useful in form-

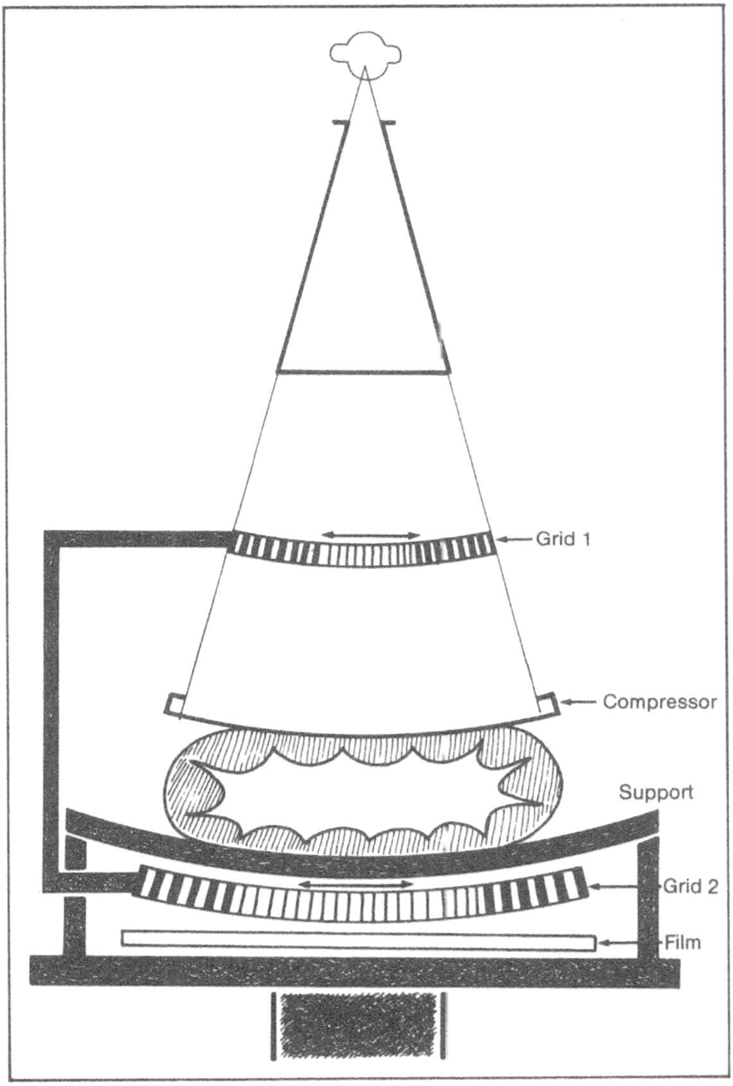

Fig. 29. Double grid unit

ing the image. As opposed to the slit unit, these grids allow for greater irradiation of the patient.

At the present time, we are experimenting with a grid made of thin, rigid metal plates without sheets. Eventually, an additional protective grid will be placed in front of the breast to prevent direct radiation from reaching the underlying plates. Additional technical problems are still being studied. While theoretically satisfactory it is still too early to reach a conclusion (Figs. 28, 29).

The Image Receiver

Film Without a Screen

Necessitating strong radiation, it provides a fine and moderately contrasted image to which mammography undoubtedly owes its rise in importance. Since it is useful, you will not find it in an antique shop, but it is gradually being abandoned.

The Film Screen Unit

Despite a slight loss in resolution the combination of a single-layer film and rare earth intensifying screen significantly reduces the irradiation and clearly reinforces the contrast.

Different speed units are marketed, with the fastest yielding slightly less definition. This diversity makes it easier to select the best compromise system since it is possible to combine different brands. Thus, one can purchase fast screens and still use slow film in the conventional manner. Decreased radiation is significant: about one-fourth the dose used for films without screens. This makes it possible to use fast film for highly opaque breasts and thus achieve the best quality.

An additional option is the use of double-emulsion industrial-type film with the screen. Theoretically, this would result in increased resolution and contrast (Frischbier).

Xerography

Here, silver-coated film is replaced by a plate coated with electrostatically charged selenium. X-rays can electrically discharge the selenium. They create a virtual image which, with a blue powder, becomes visible (Figs. 30, 31). Compared with mammography, xerography is easier to use for several reasons:

- Good-quality images can be produced by nonspecialized radiologic equipment.
- Compression is not indispensable.
- Interpretation of the images is easy.

With the present-day technique, however, a xerographic image provides less information than a good mammogram on conventional film. Compare the two under a magnifying glass. Because of its grain, xerography does not withstand the test whereas conventional film will show small detail. As for the contrast it is true that at first glance it appears to be of high quality at all levels in xerography. If strong correct lighting of variable intensity is used, however, the same excellent contrast will be seen on conventional film.

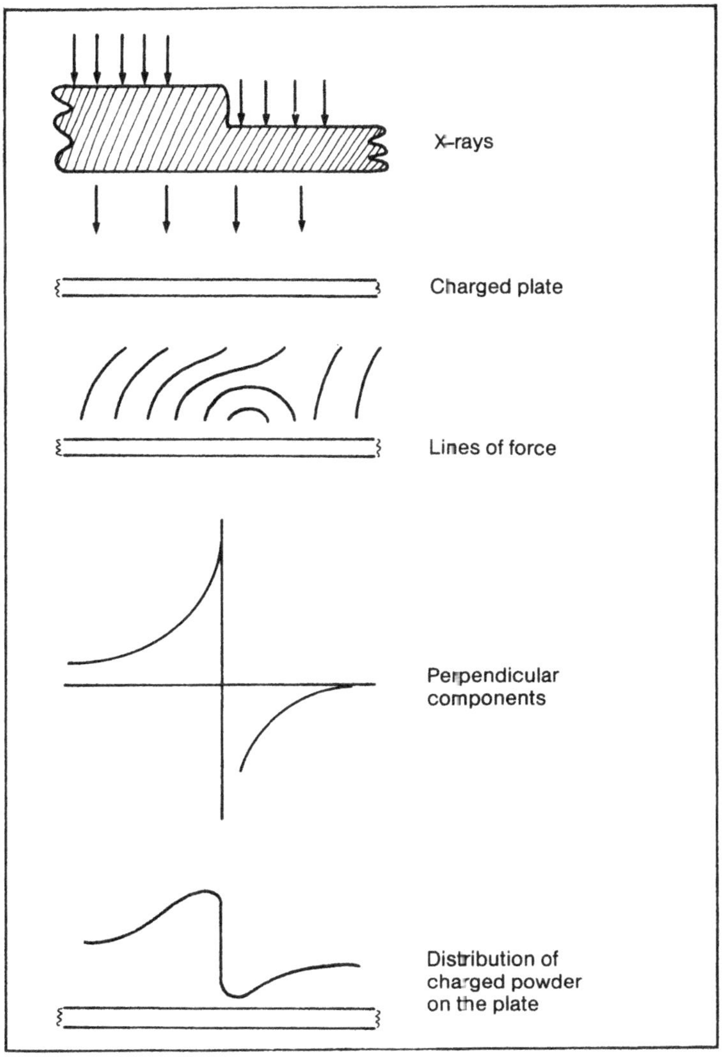

Fig. 30. Xerography: contour-reinforcement. (From "Technical application" Bulletin 1, Nov. 1974, Xerox Corporation)

Xerography does make it possible to obtain a global view extending beyond the limits of the compressed breast. The axillary region and chest wall are clearly visible. This is particularly valuable in pre- and post-therapeutic examinations for carcinoma. It is difficult to compare radiation doses of the two methods because of the different voltages used. There appears to be more irradiation with xerography than with mammography for the film-screen units and less for film alone.

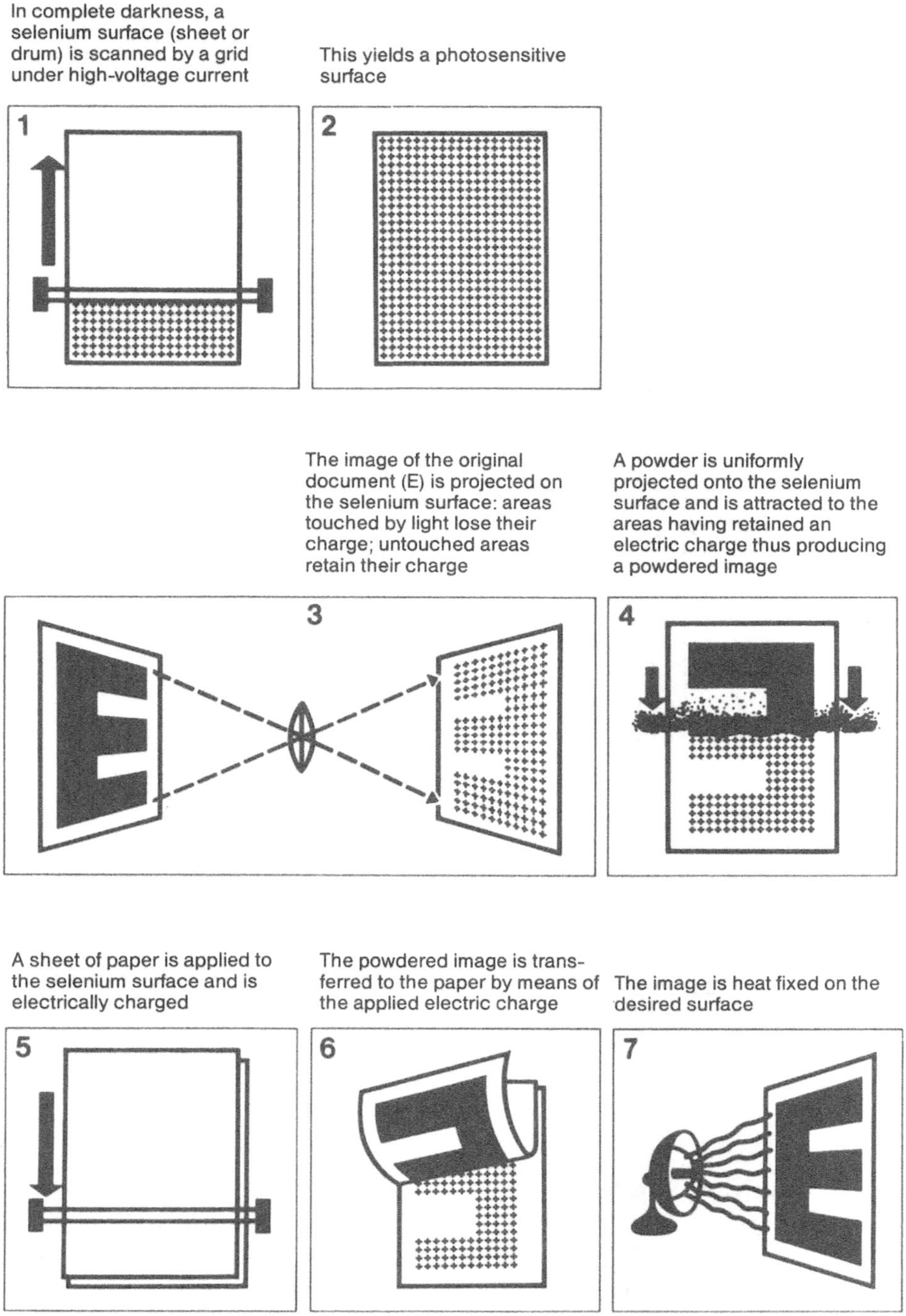

Fig. 31. Xerography (Doc. Rank Xerox)

Ionography

This technique uses the effect of X-rays on gaseous ions. While still in the research stage it has already provided some very interesting films with respect to contrast and resolution.

Film Development

Originally, films without the screen had to be developed by hand.

Emulsions were then developed which could undergo machine treatment, at first in a slow cycle: 8 min, then 3.5 min, and finally 1.5 min. Results obtained with a fast cycle were comparable to those obtained slowly by machine or manually. Monolayer films printed with the screen are easily developed in the fast cycle. It is essential that the material be in good condition and clean in order to avoid artifacts.

Fluorescent Scope

The choice of equipment for reading the films is far from secondary. The scope should be able to fit at least six 18 × 24 cm films simultaneously. A powerful spot light as well as a strong magnifying glass should always be available.

Undoubtedly, physicists could explain to us why a cloudless sky is the best of scopes. This is particularly true for complex mammograms which appear to have many more images when seen through this natural light.

Fluoroscopy

Fluoroscopy of the breast is not currently used but could and will be, thanks to amplification. It will be useful for the localisation and puncture of nonpalpable lesions.

1.5.1.3 Technique

Positioning

Except under certain circumstances, the examination is bilateral. Three views are used for each breast:

- Craniocaudal (Fig. 32)
- Lateromedial (Fig. 33)
- Oblique (covering the axillary part of the breast) (Fig. 34)

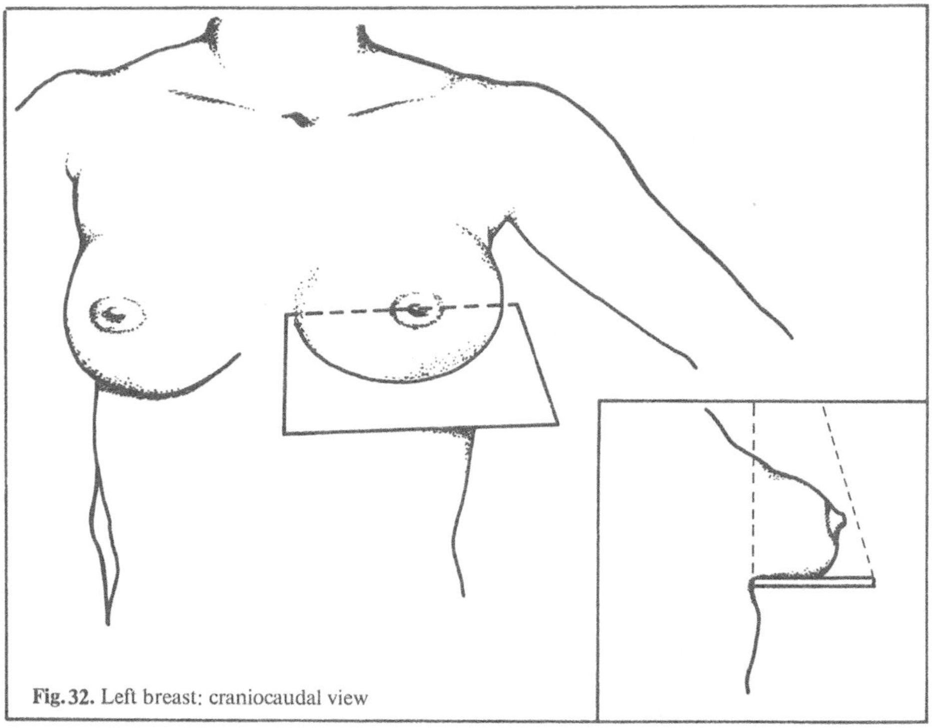

Fig. 32. Left breast: craniocaudal view

As much of the mammary tissue as possible should be included on the film for each view, as well as the nipple, which should be imaged tangentially without distortion. This makes for less superimposition of lactiferous elements and connective tissue bands and for fewer artifacts.

By flattening and evenly distributing the breast tissue, compression reduces the penetration necessary. This should be done firmly but gently. Being able to assure the patient and gain her confidence has an important soothing effect.

The patient is seated for the examination (stands for certain adjustments).

Craniocaudal view: Without raising her shoulder, the patient places her hand on the hip ipsilateral to the side being imaged. The breast rests on a small examining table. The submammary fold is brought up to the level of the table by adjusting the latter or the seat. Compression is progressively applied while the radiologist, standing behind the patient, holds the breast in place and pulls it forward until the last second. A flat ruler can be used instead of the hand for very small breasts.

Lateromedial view: The patient raises her arm up on the side to be imaged. The radiologist stands on the other side and places the breast in position, taking in as much of the medial border skin as possible. Compression should not offset the nipple.

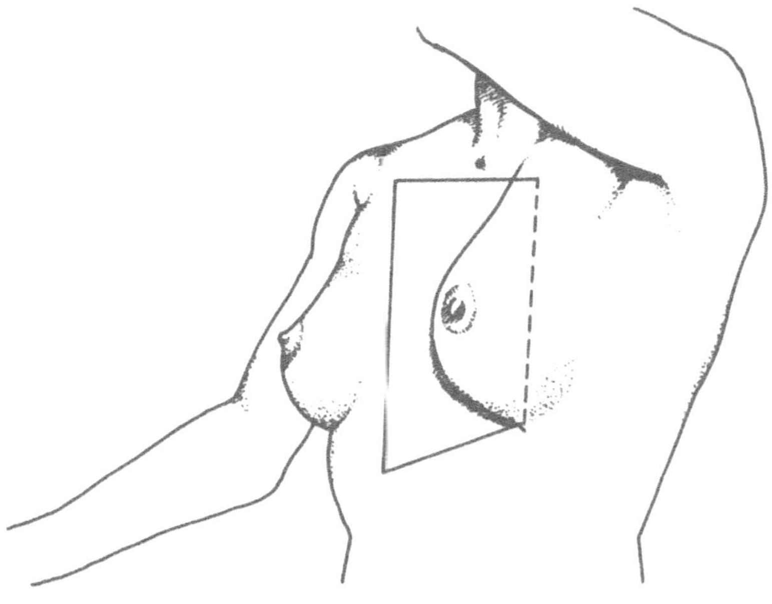

Fig. 33. Left breast: lateromedial view

Oblique view: The table is angled 30–60° in a vertical plane according to the patient's build (greater angle for thinner subjects). The lateral aspect of the breast is placed against the table. The radiologist takes the axillary portion of the breast together with the pectoral muscle and places them against the table in such a way that the sensitive surface on the table moves along with it and lodges in the axilla.

Pressure must be applied gently and only to the breast. If the patient is sitting too low, compression will involve the shoulder and, thus, will be painful and less effective.

Special views: These are often less useful than is generally believed. In certain cases, however, it may be necessary to image a lesion tangentially or use a lateral profile view to study a difficult image.

A special lateral view in xerography places the patient in an oblique supine position, turned toward the side to be imaged. Highly radiotranslucent cushions keep the breast in the correct sagittal position.

Enlargement: Geometric enlargement occurs when the distance between the film and patient increases. Resolution is better since the grain of the film-screen unit becomes negligible and part of the secondary radiation does not reach the

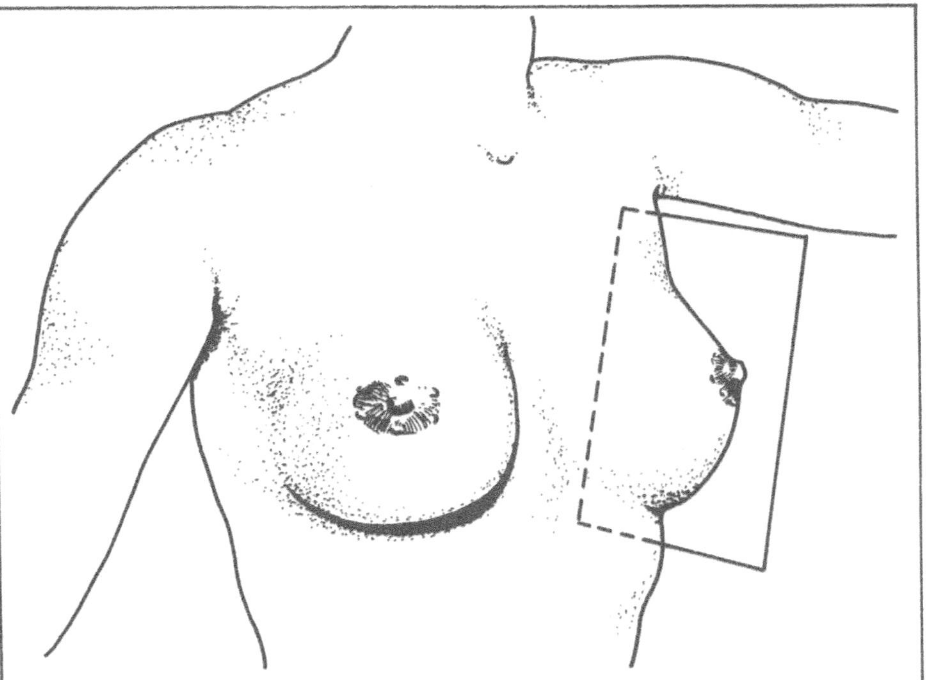

Fig. 34. Left breast: oblique view

film. Size of the focal spot is, however, a limiting factor. For an enlargement of 1.5, the focal spot cannot exceed 0.3 mm (Fig. 35).

A disadvantage of enlargement is the decrease in contrasts. Small, poorly contrasted details may go undetected.

Technical Parameters

It is impossible to talk about numbers here considering the many differences between units. What is important is establishing the principles for adapting the technique to variations in breast opacity.

The average breast: Let us take as an example a breast measuring 3 cm under compression with 50% adipose tissue as shown by the film.

The basic technical sequence includes:

- Molybdenum anode
- Beryllium window
- Molybdenum filter
- 28 kV in monophase
- Slow single layer film with fast rare earth screen
- Machine development in 90 s

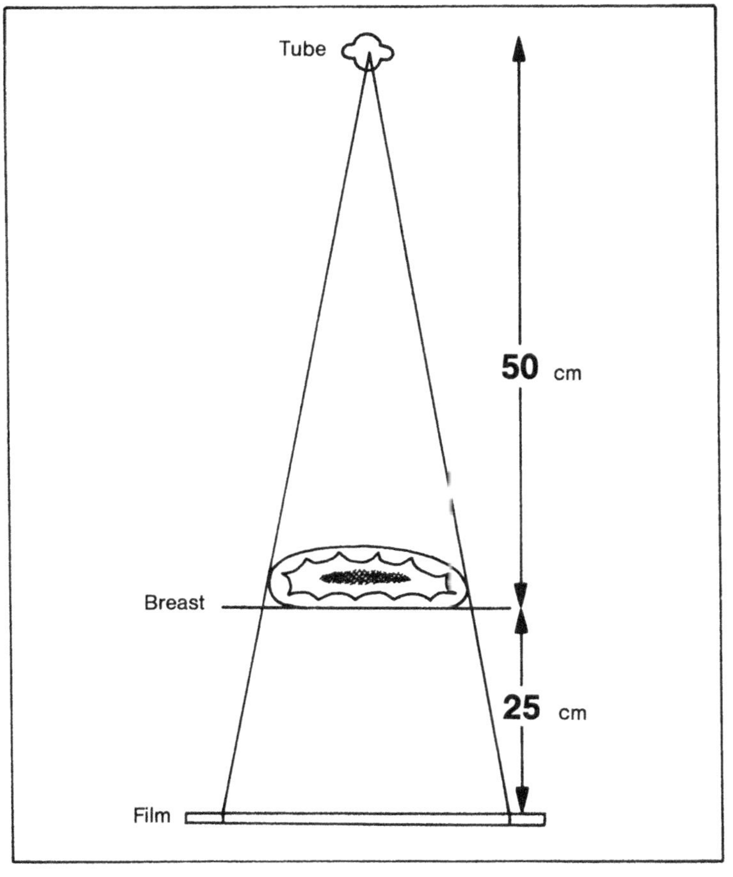

Fig. 35. Direct enlargement technique

The transparent breast (very slight or highly adipose): By lowering the coefficients, the same technical sequence can be used. It is best not to go below 25 kV so adjustments will be made by varying the milliamperage. While film alone, or with the slow screen, can be used, there is no strong argument to justify this technical diversification.

The opaque breast (very opaque or very dense): For the slightly more opaque than average breast to the highly opaque breast, we feel the best opinions are as follows:

- Passage from slow to fast film
- Coefficients increased to 30 kV, 200 mA
- 0.5-mm aluminum instead of 0.03-mm molybdenum filter

  In each case, the film is correctly darkened but image contrast is often poor. Results can be improved by two different techniques:
- Use of a grid (see above)

- Direct film duplication. This special contact film produces a negative from a negative.

In order to obtain an exact reproduction, exposure must occur in ultraviolet light. If white light is used, the contrast is greatly increased. Exposure times vary with the type of flash used. By increasing the exposure, we reduce the darkening of the reproduction and vice versa.

It is convenient and economical to use the light field of an inexpensive photocopier. The film to be duplicated is placed on the field; the negative is placed on top, dull (emulsion) side down. Development takes place in 90 s with a fast machine.

1.5.1.4 Interpretation of the Overall Structure

Total density of the breast: This is certainly an important factor and can be immediately determined providing the technical conditions of the procedure are known. It depends on the degree of penetration. The two significant extremes are:

- The highly transparent breast, clearly adipose with no active glandular tissue
- The highly opaque breast, which is active and to which excess hydration and cellular proliferation is added

The importance of contrast:

When the entire breast is transparent, the slightest image, be it normal (fibroglandular bands, vessels) or pathologic (tumors, calcification), will be well contrasted.

When the breast is dense it is best to try to determine the type of image according to those elements which can be identified:

- Functional excess hydration is highly dense with few contrasts and few visible images (Fig. 36).
- Mastosic proliferation has many fibronodular type images which are more or less distinct depending on the degree of stromal hydration. The overall image may be either predominantly fibrous or nodular (Fig. 37).
- The combination of functional excess and mastosic proliferation is usually the case. However, it is often possible to determine a predominance of one or the other:
  Fibrous elements (Fig. 38)
  Fibroadipose elements (Fig. 39)
  Fibromicronodular elements (1- to 2-mm nodules) (Fig. 40)
  Fibromacronodular elements (nodules greater than 4 mm) (Fig. 41)
  Fibroheteronodular elements (Fig. 42)
- Tissular characteristics may be homogeneous or scattered in patches. Normal involution first occurs in the inner and lower quadrants leaving active tissue along with its axillary projections in the upper-outer quadrants.

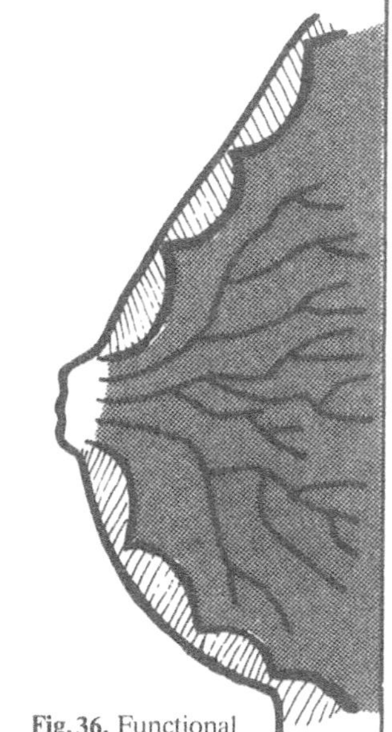
Fig. 36. Functional excess hydration

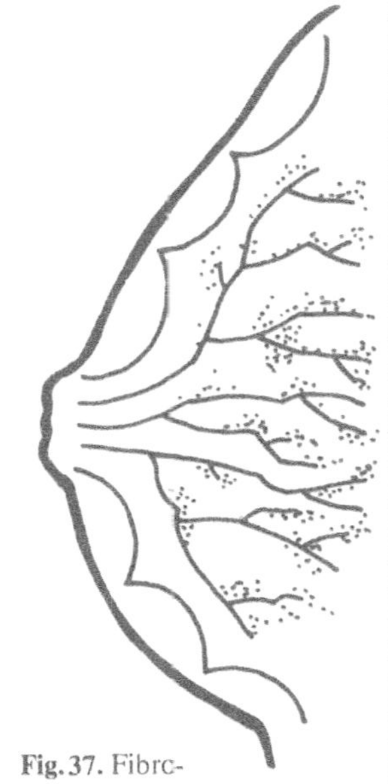
Fig. 37. Fibro-nodular mastosis

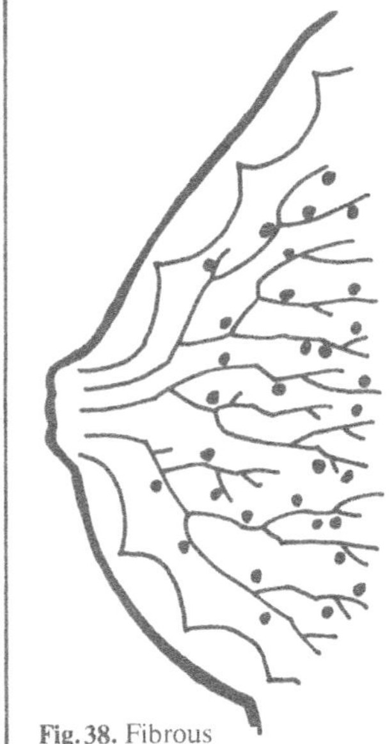
Fig. 38. Fibrous elements

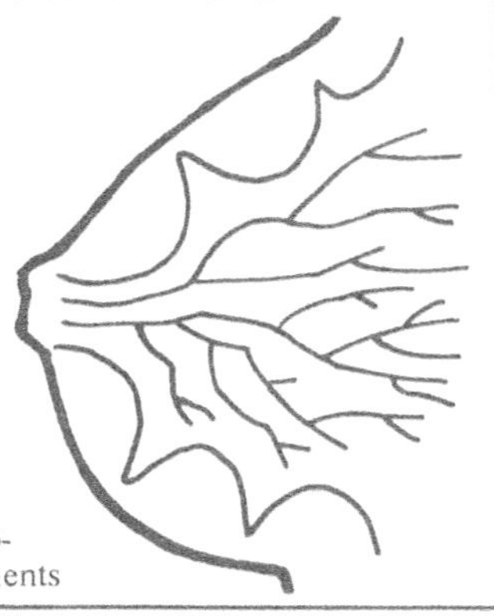
Fig. 39. Fibro-adipose elements

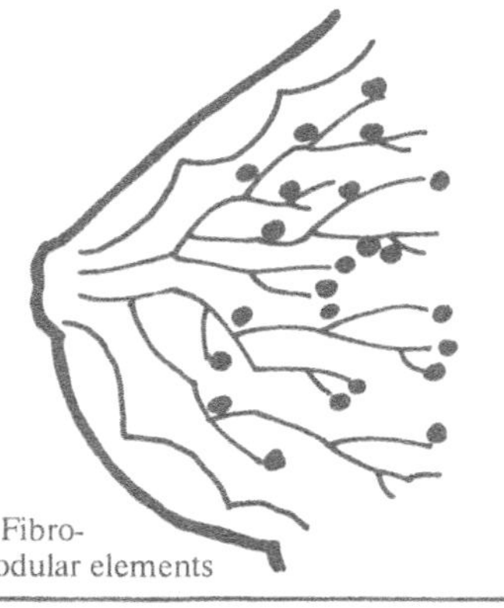
Fig. 40. Fibro-micronodular elements

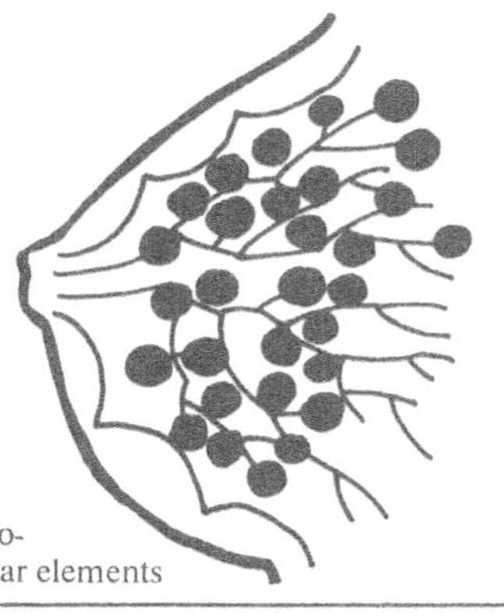
Fig. 41. Fibro-macronodular elements

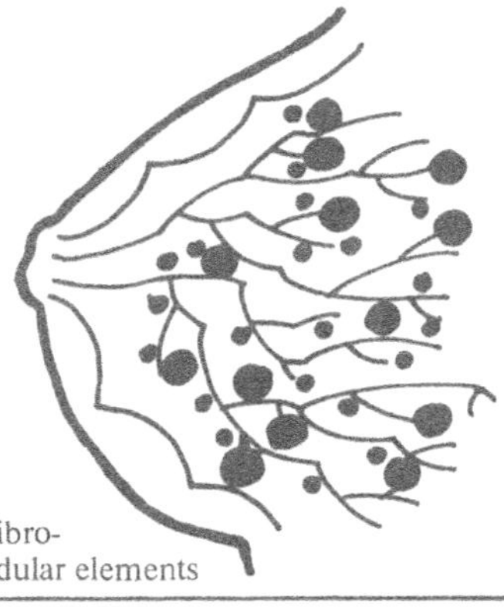
Fig. 42. Fibro-heteronodular elements

1.5.1.5 Interpretation of Abnormalities

The Skin

Thickening Corresponds to Edematous Infiltration

- Localized: superficial or deep mastitis, subareolar abscess, Mondor's disease, superficial neoplasia (Fig. 43)
- Diffuse: inflammatory carcinoma, acute mastitis, radiation sequelae (Fig. 44)

Retraction

The tangenital view of the breast's cutaneous outline is depressed. Subcutaneous tissue below, contains fine bands fixing the skin to the gland or to an underlying lesion.

If this abnormality is not seen tangentially, it forms a linear opacity like a skin fold (Fig. 45).

This retraction is characteristic of carcinoma but may also represent a surgical scar or sequelae of Mondor's disease.

Subcutaneous Adipose Tissue

If it develops at the surface, a clearly delineated structure (cyst, fibroadenoma, phylloide tumor, sarcoma) flattens the subcutaneous adipose tissue to a fine transparent line (Fig. 46). Local infiltration of carcinoma may cause changes in the subcutaneous adipose tissue: decrease, densification, opacities of the tumor itself (Fig. 47).

The Mammary Gland

Mammogram Hypertranslucency

Two elements are more translucent than the average glandular tissue: air and fat.

Air Translucency
Artificial contrast of cystography will be discussed later. The only spontaneously occurring gaseous contrast is the air galactogram: air filling 2–3 cm of one or several lactiferous ducts, generally in the retroareolar area, provides excellent contrast (Fig. 48).

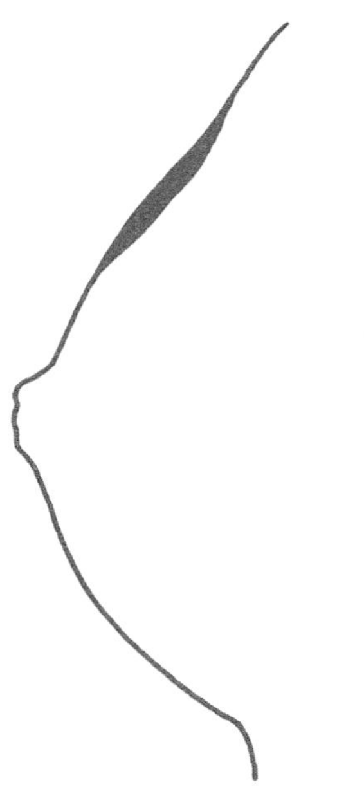

Fig. 43. Localized thickening

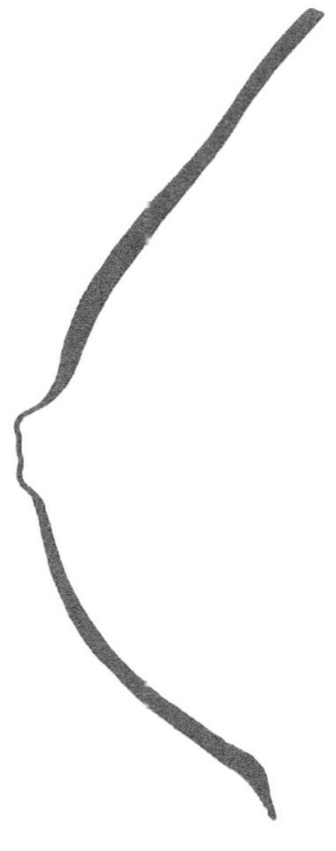

Fig. 44. Overall thickening

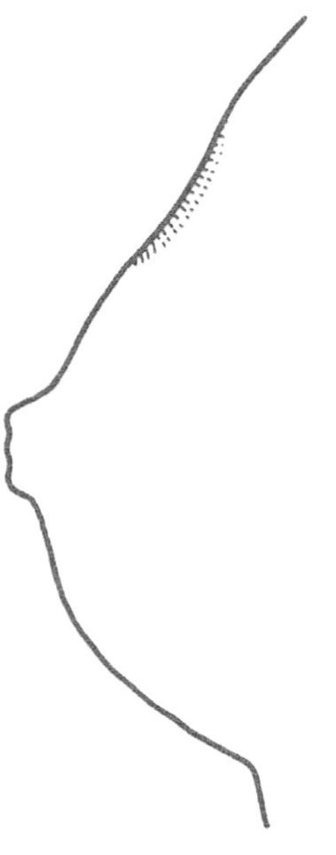

Fig. 45. Skin retraction

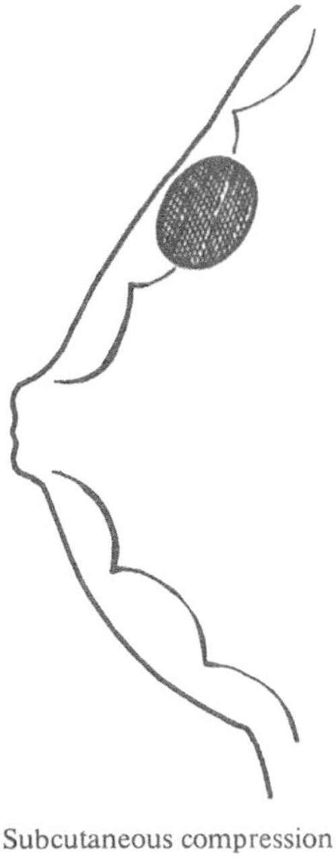

Fig. 46. Subcutaneous compression by a mass

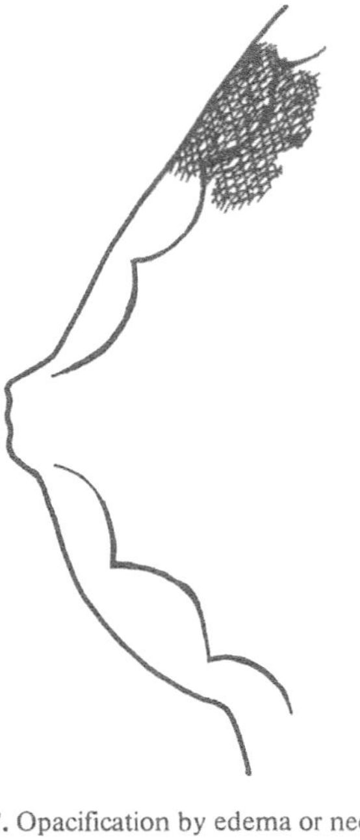

Fig. 47. Opacification by edema or neoplastic process

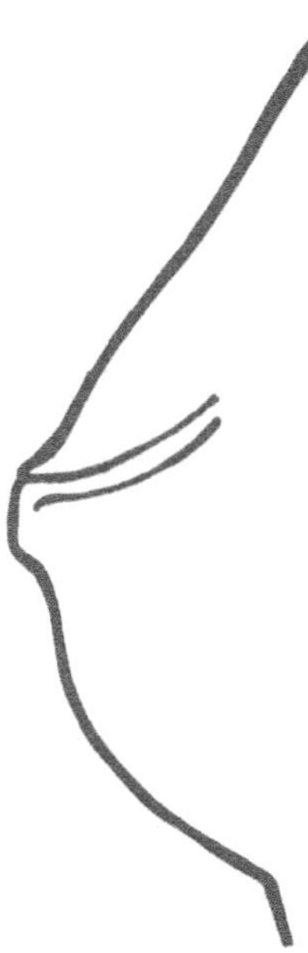

Fig. 48. Ductal air translucency

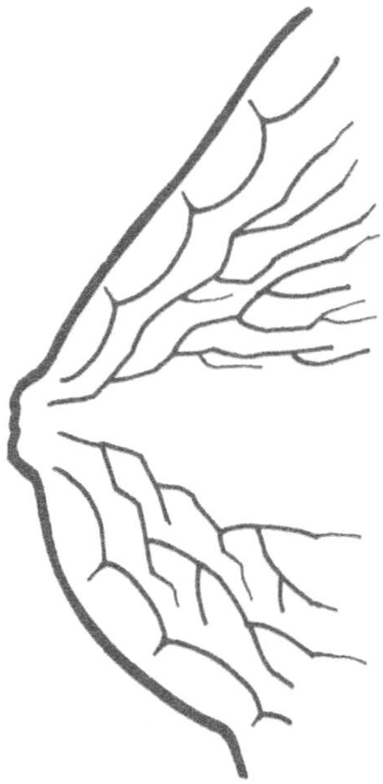

Fig. 49. Adipose translucency

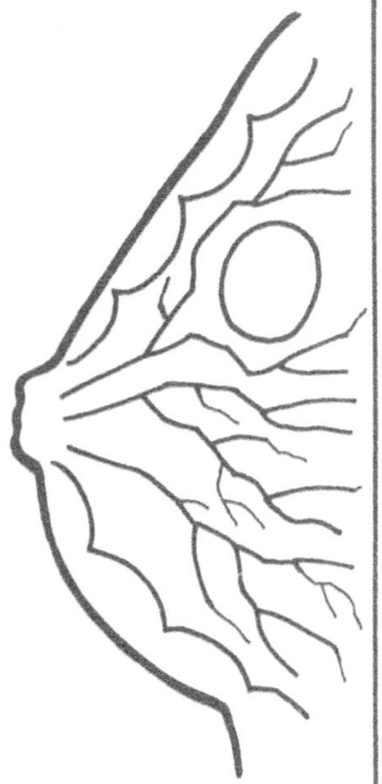

Fig. 50. Oil cyst

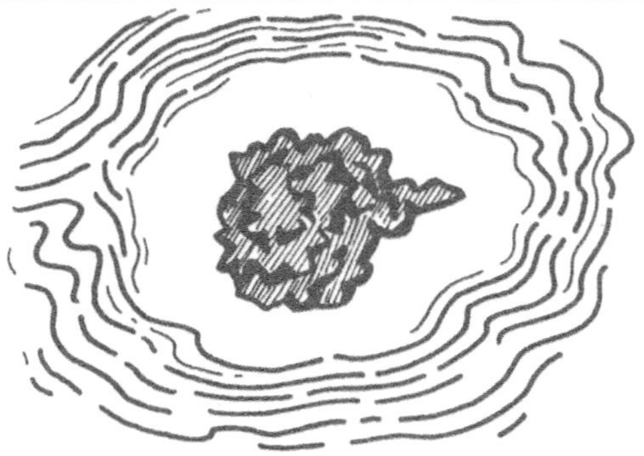

Fig. 51. Nodule. Signs of malignancy:
- Radioclinical dissociation: the radiographic nodule is smaller than the palpated mass
- Irregular form
- Poorly delineated contour covered with spicules
- Heterogeneous
- Change in surrounding tissue: clear halo or condensation
- Microcalcification

Adipose Translucency
Most often, these are relatively localized fatty patches. Since unencapsulated, they are not well defined. This is not a pathologic image (Fig. 49).

Occasionally a fatty translucency will be surrounded by a capsule (Fig. 50). This may occur in common lipomas. Fat necrosis may occur after trauma or surgery with the macroscopic appearance of a "lipid cyst." Galactocele erosion may produce an oil cyst: the opaque milky fluid gives the galactocele the radiographic density of a benign cyst. Lipid transformation gives it a fatty hypertranslucency.

Mammogram Hyperdensities

Three types of images can be described: nodules, opaque patches, and abnormal bands.

1. Because of its contour and/or density a nodule is well delineated.

- Positive diagnosis: confirm the presence of the nodule. This may be easy with an unobstructed mammogram. It is sometimes more difficult with a fibronodular breast in which a slightly denser, more distinct, larger image can only be relatively distinguished.
- Differential diagnosis: A displaced nipple may appear as a false nodule. False nodular images due to cutaneous lesions or lymph nodes are more difficult to identify.

Description

- Size: from 1 mm to several centimeters in diameter. Over 4 cm is considered a mass. It is important to indicate if the size of the visible nodule is the same or less than that of the palpated nodule
- Site: according to the classic quadrants and also according to depth
- Form: round, oval, polycyclic
- Contour: distinct or blurred, smooth or spicular, uninterrupted or fragmented
- Structure: homogeneous or heterogeneous, degree of density, with or without calcifications
- Surrounding tissue: unaffected or modified, more opaque or more translucent

Significance

The radiologic nodular image is found in many benign and malignant breast diseases. Detection of a nodule requires a formal diagnosis often needing cytologic or histologic confirmation. Other radiologic characteristics of each disease are equally valuable for orienting the diagnosis. These are discussed in the chapters on breast disease: cyst, fibroadenoma, adenoma, phylloide tumor, abscess, hemorrhagic cyst, hemangioma, etc. There is no pathognomonic sign of the benign nature of a nodule. In other words, any nodule may represent carcinoma. Obviously this does not mean that all mammographic nodules should be considered as carcinoma. It does mean that the criteria of the benign nature of a nodular radiographic opacity are only accessory findings and in no way should counter evidence of malignancy demonstrated by another method. For example, a mammographic nodule in an area where thermography shows hyperthermia should be considered suspect whatever the radiologic appearance.

For this reason, we will not describe what are commonly called the criteria of benign lesions. It is important, however, to consider the signs of malignancy, each of which is reason for concern (Fig. 51).

- The radiographic nodule is smaller than the palpated nodule (since the hand cannot distinguish between the lesion itself and the peritumoral induration that occurs with carcinoma):

- It has an irregular form
- Poorly deliniated contour, covered with spicules
- Heterogeneous structure with areas of high density
- Diffuse modification in the transparency of the surrounding tissues: either edematous condensation or hypertranslucency due to the peritumoral fat which is compressed
- Associated signs: cutaneous and subcutaneous changes, microcalcification.

Multiple nodules may represent multiple sites of the same disease. When spread over a large area or even the entire breast, the nodule may enter into the description of the type of tissue (dystrophic nodules, microcysts).

2. The opaque patch is an area characterized simply by its density, which is greater than that of the rest of the breast. It has neither the nodule's form nor its contour. This image may appear in four circumstances:

- The area in question contains normal glandular tissue but contrasts with adipose involution of the surrounding tissue. Even more frequently, the image is due to increased thickness related to the breast's morphology or its position during the examination. In the latter case, the opaque patch is not found in all views (Fig. 52).
- The area in question is the site of an actual increase in opacity corresponding to an edematous process: common inflammation, trauma, estrogen hyperactivity (Fig. 53).
- The area in question is the site of a dystrophic process. Condensation is due to cellular proliferation (adenosis), sclerosis, and edema (Fig. 54).
- The area in question is the site of carcinoma: there is no distinguishable nodule. The opacity may be due to the cell multiplication as well as the edema (Fig. 55).

In each of these four cases, the physical principle for formation of the patch is the same: cellular density and water. This image in itself, therefore, cannot be formal evidence in favour of a benign or malignant nature. Certain signs can help to determine its origin.

The appearance is somewhere between that of a nodule and diffuse tissue change. Signs that are similar to those characterizing a nodule tend to give the patch greater pathologic significance. Consequently, the less diffuse the image, the greater its opacity and the more it merits consideration.

Associated radiologic abnormalities may be of major importance: fibrous bands, microcalcification. Identifying the abnormality says nothing about its benign or malignant nature. This is well illustrated by the difficulty in the diagnosis of sclerosing adenosis. Only a thorough study by the pathologist will differentiate it from carcinoma.

Within certain limits, we can use evolutive criteria. Providing there is no indication for immediate action, image stability or its regression under medical treatment is generally considered evidence of its benign nature. Carcinoma,

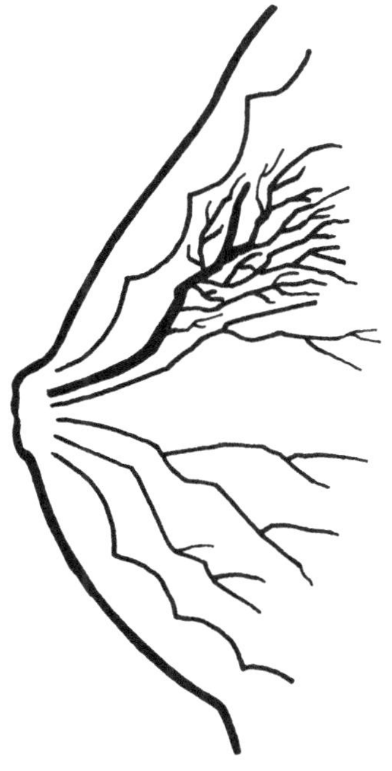

Fig. 52. Effect of glandular and adipose distribution

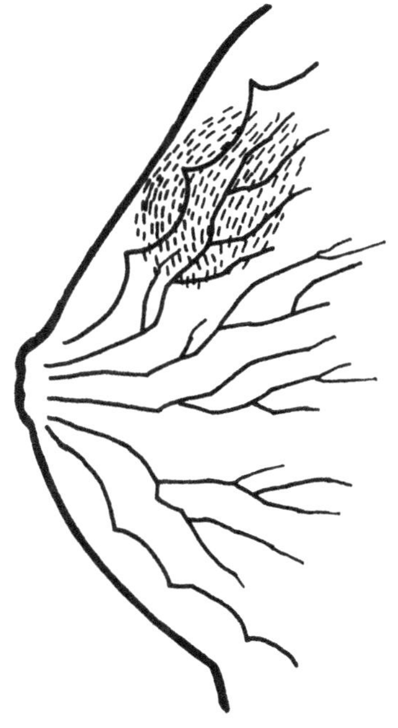

Fig. 53. Localized edema

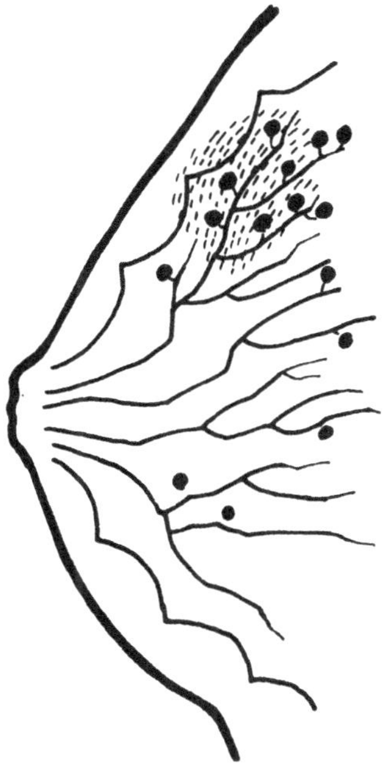

Fig. 54. Dystrophy

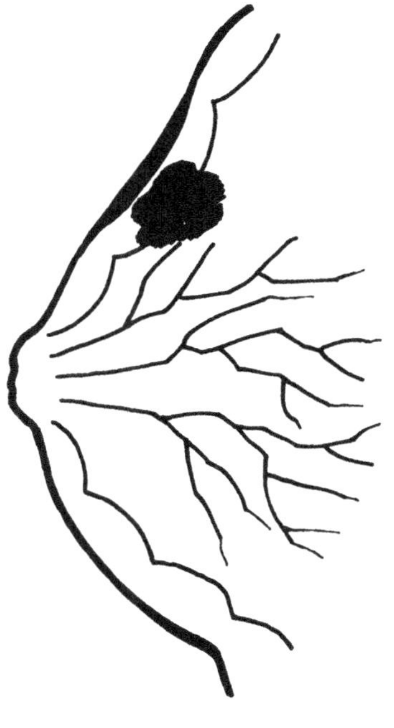

Fig. 55. Carcinoma

however, may also have periods of spontaneous stabilization. Even a decrease in peritumoral edema may simulate regression of the lesion.

3. Abnormal bands may suggest striae (Fig. 56), tractus (Fig. 57), and spicules (Fig. 58). Opaque lines of variable thickness and length are part of the normal mammogram. They correspond to branchings of connective tissue and lactiferous elements which project to the skin into Duret's crests. These bands, adjacent to pathologic images or without apparent cause, may undergo change which can be detected by comparison with the general structure of the examined breast:

- Unusual direction, neither toward the nipple nor toward a crest
- Abnormally high number of tightly packed striae
- Excessive thickness and/or density of these images
- Especially, projection of these images toward an abnormality: pathologic nodular opacity, cutaneous thickening

Pathologic linear images represent sclerosing processes. They may develop after surgery, trauma, and infection. They are also seen in dystrophic diseases. Their detection is particularly valuable in neoplastic diseases where they correspond to the perilesional stroma reaction. They form the peritumoral spiculations, both short and long, and account for cutaneous and nipple retraction. These fibrous-appearing bands may contain neoplastic elements and, thus, should be considered as part of the lesion when determining tumor size.

The stellate image (Fig. 59) is a particular type of linear appearance. Convergence of the bands may be only a result of superimposition. This can be confirmed by comparing several different views. A true dense stellate image corresponds to early carcinoma in 80% of cases. But, the diagnosis may be difficult considering other processes have similar appearances:

- Sclerosing adenosis
- Post-traumatic fibrosis
- Surgical scar
- Acute mastitis

Calcifications

Calcifications of the breast differ from all other abnormal hyperdensities by the high atomic mass of calcium which results in intense radiologic opacity even for small sizes. In order for a microcalcification to be visible on the film, however, the shadow it casts must not be too large. As the shadow increases, its density decreases and it may not create sufficient contrast. This explains the importance of geometric conditions in constructing the image: focal spot dimensions, focal spot-film distance, grain of the screen and film.

1. The nature of some calcifications is evident:

- Thick arciform calcifications of an old fibroadenoma (Fig. 60), fine, more or less spherical, calcifications of a cyst or fat necrosis (Fig. 61)

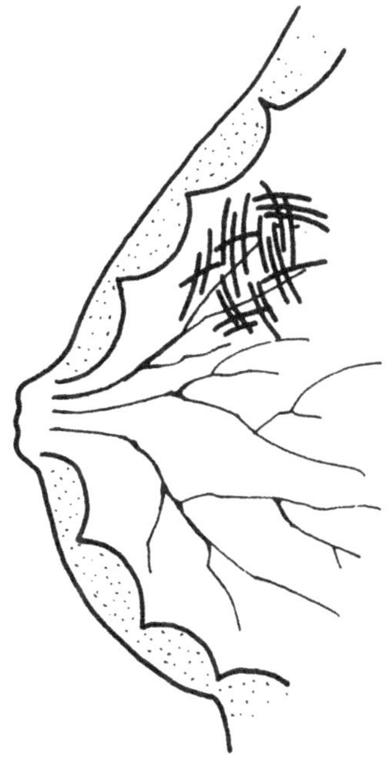

Fig. 56. Striae

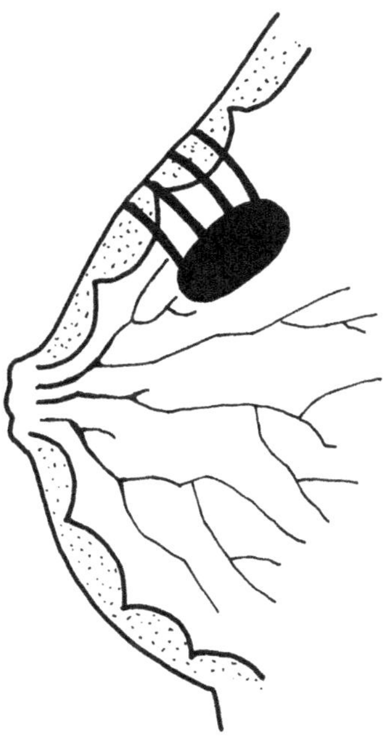

Fig. 57. Tractus

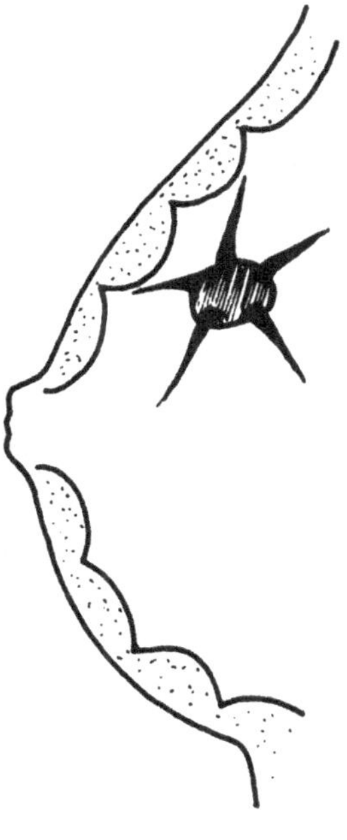

Fig. 58. Spicules

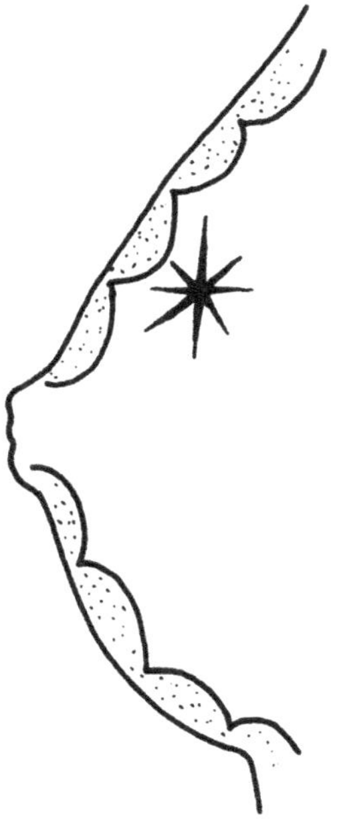

Fig. 59. Stellate image

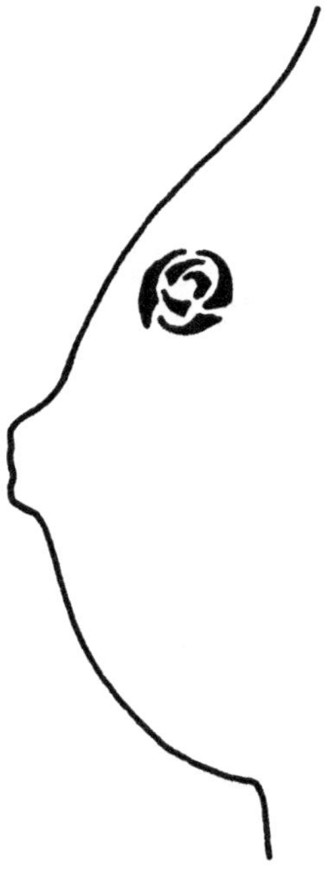

Fig. 60. Calcified fibroadenoma

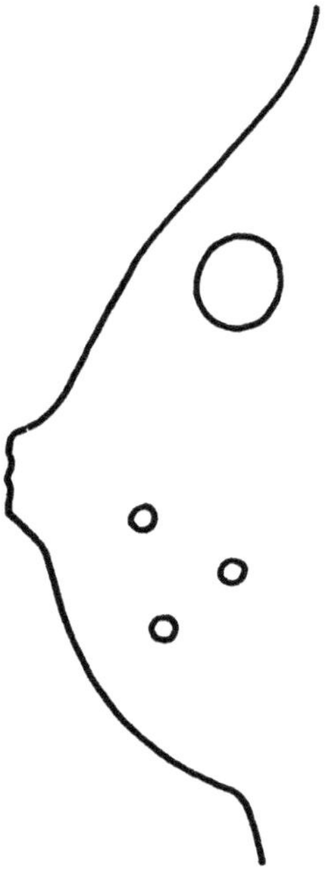

Fig. 61. Cystic calcifications and fat necrosis

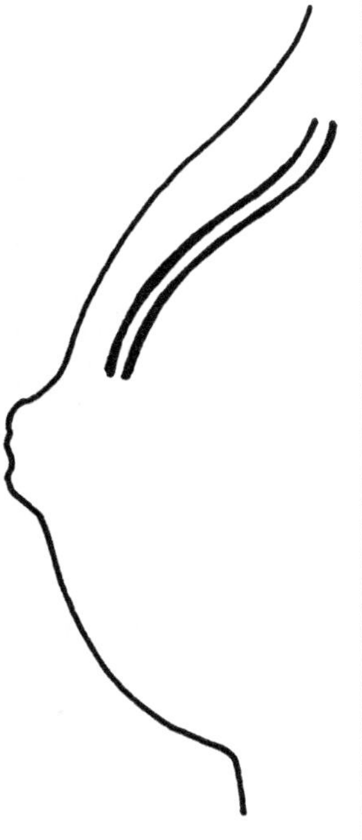

Fig. 62. Vascular calcification

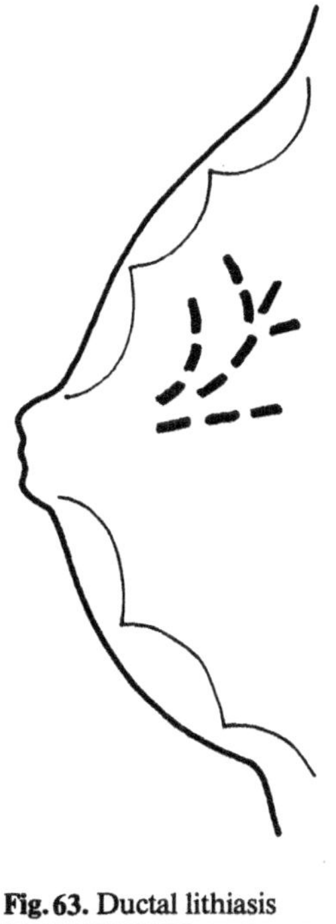

Fig. 63. Ductal lithiasis

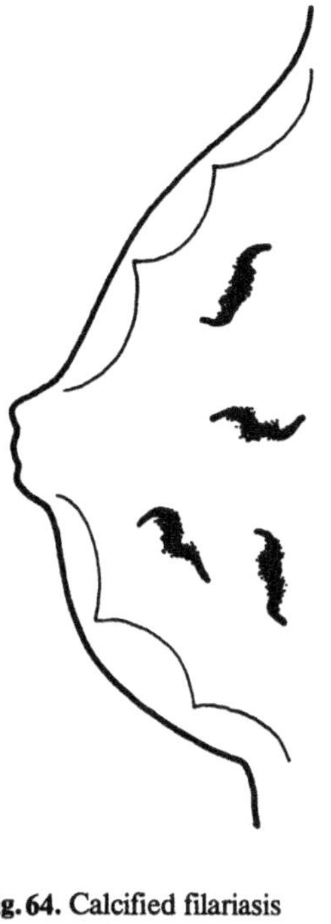

Fig. 64. Calcified filariasis

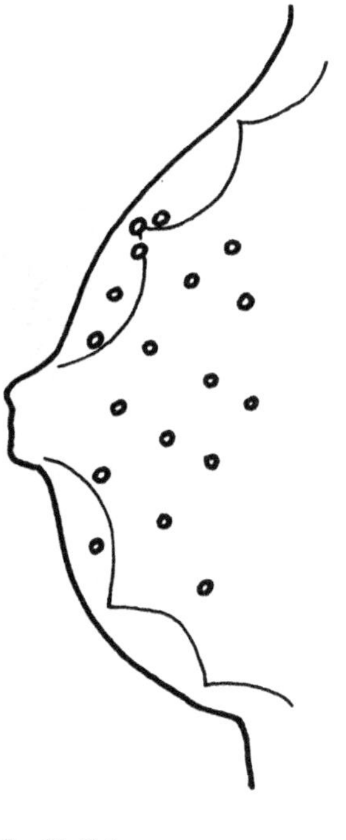

Fig. 65. Talc

- Vascular calcifications which are sinuous bands with sharp borders and somewhat bumpy surfaces (Fig. 62)
- Ductal lithiasis in the form of rods along the ductal axes (Fig. 63)
- Three-centimeter-long sinuous, linear calcifications of the filariasis only rarely observed in Africa (Fig. 64)
- Superficial, diffuse, round millicalcifications in the skin observed in a tangential view due to repeated use of talc (Fig. 65)

2. All other calcifications may be problematic.

Calcification is a late response to tissue injury for many processes: trauma, infection, and dystrophy are all as apt as cancer to create such images. While it may be possible to describe certain characteristic aspects in order to differentiate between some of these processes, the conditions under which the image is constructed must be taken into account.

Once again, visualization of a microcalcification depends on the technical conditions of the examination. Thus, calcifications are just one factor in orienting the diagnosis for comedocarcinoma (Fig. 66), nodular or hard carcinoma (Fig. 67), mastosis – described in later chapters – and plasma cell mastitis (Fig. 68).

The importance of the distribution of the calcifications should be stressed. If located in one particular area, they may be determinant in fixing the site of needle aspiration or deciding to biopsy. When diffuse and only slightly contrasted they most often correspond to common mastosis (Fig. 69) but may also be found in lobular carcinoma (Fig. 70).

Vascular Images

Vascular images may be visible in a radiolucent breast and in subcutaneous adipose tissue. These are superficial veins whose diameter should be determined (Fig. 71). Varicose ectasia may occur. It is particularly interesting to look for an increase in diameter of veins adjacent to a lesion. When increased by a factor of 1.5 (as compared with the other side), this is an indirect sign in favor of cancer.

Lymph Node Opacities

Lymph node opacities may be included in a descriptive illustration, but do they provide any useful information for the diagnosis? This is rarely the case, and those images characteristic of cancerous nodes: large volume, high density, blurred or spiculated contours are easily palpated lesions (Fig. 73). The image of a node with sharp contours and a light center (Fig. 72) is no more an indication of its benign nature than the absence of medullary radiolucence signals malignancy. Occasionally, however, the radiographic image of adenopathy may be cause to double check a hasty palpation.

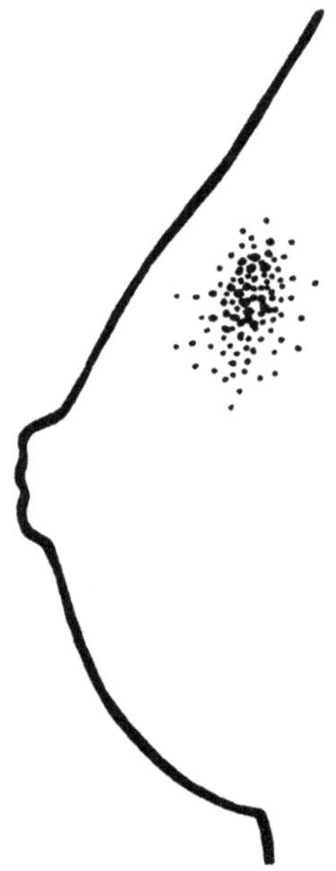

Fig. 66. Comedocarcinoma

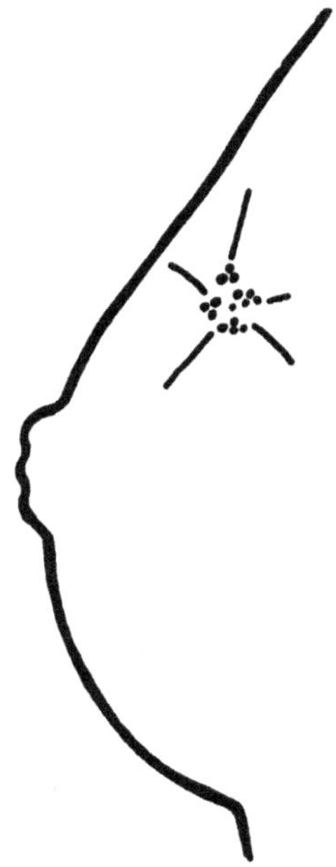

Fig. 67. Microcalcifications in scirrhous or nodular carcinoma

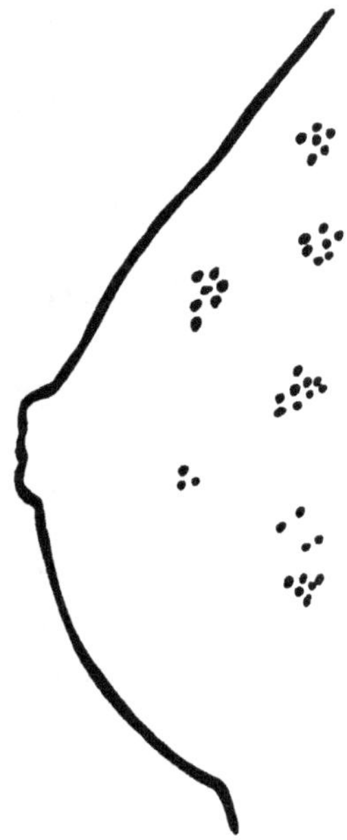

Fig. 70. Diffuse microcalcifications of lobular carcinoma

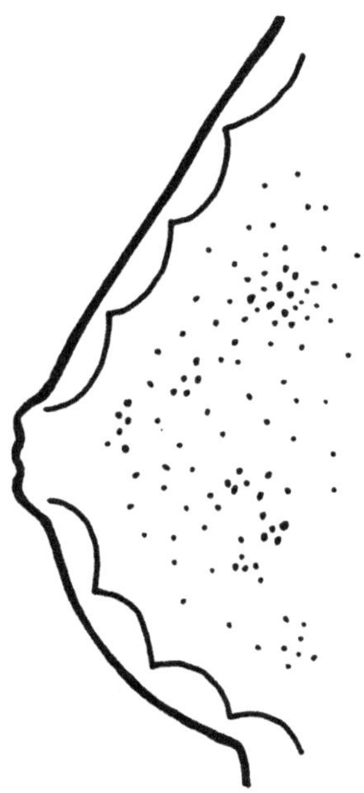

Fig. 69. Mastosic calcifications

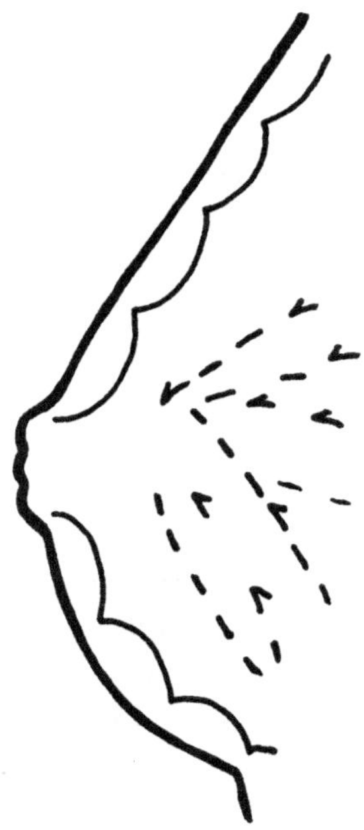

Fig. 68. Microcalcifications of plasma-cell mastitis

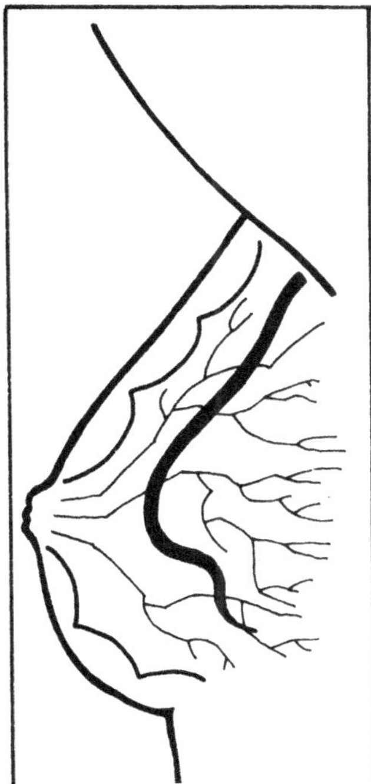

Fig. 71. Vascular images: distinctly visible vein in a fatty breast

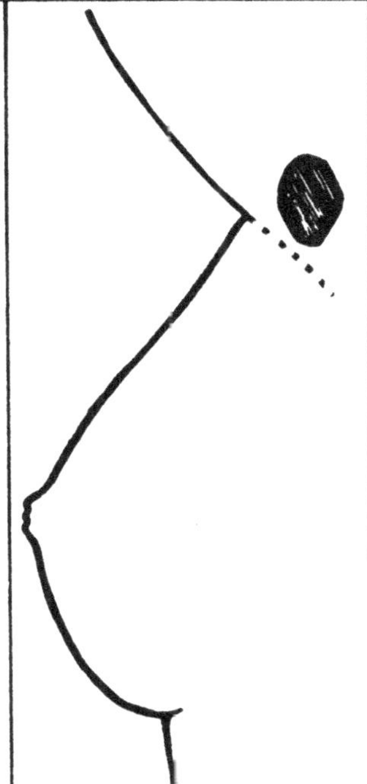

Fig. 72. Lymph node opacities: benign lymph node

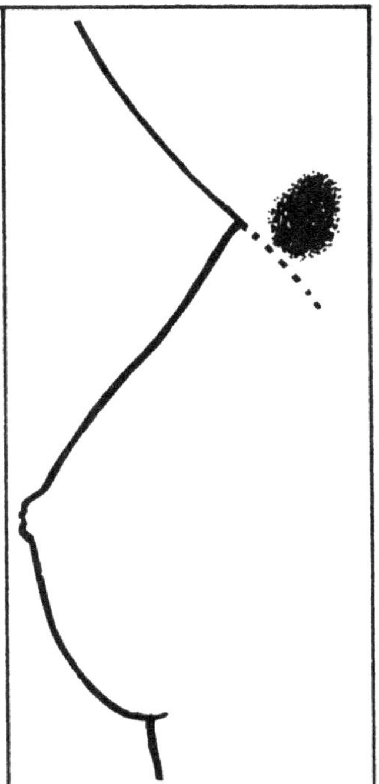

Fig. 73. Lymph node opacities: malignant lymph node

Strong Points

- Adipose or slightly hydrated breasts
- Neoplastic lesions, even if small or deep

Weak Points

- Breasts with excess hydration
- Mastosis
- Fluid cavity detection

1.5.2 Galactography

1.5.2.1 Technique

This is mammography following lactiferous duct opacification through its nipple aperture. It is difficult to perform if the duct is not spontaneously dilated. Generally, however, dilation occurs with discharge.

The patient is in the inclined or supine position. The surface of the nipple is always first cleaned and disinfected (Mercryl). A 2%–5% Novocain-soaked

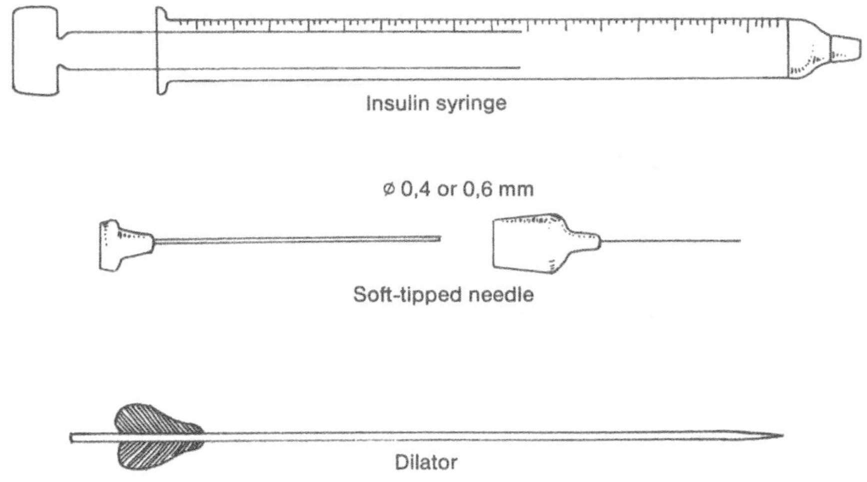

Fig. 74. Galactography: material

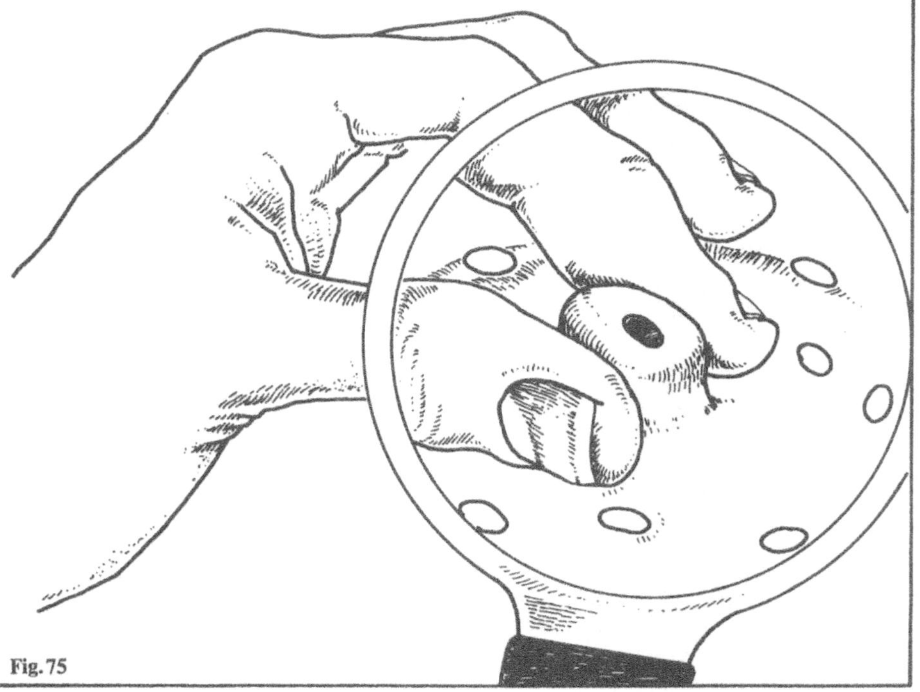

Fig. 75

compress can be briefly applied to the nipple in order to facilitate catheterization and provide less discomfort for the patient. The oozing lactiferous duct can be located through a magnifying-glass by compressing the areola or the entire breast (Fig. 75).

The dilator is a fine, soft-tipped conical instrument (Fig. 74). It is gently inserted into the duct and held for 1 or 2 min with increasing pressure and slight circular movements (Fig. 76). An insulin syringe and high gauge (0.4 or 0.6 mm), soft-tipped needle are used for injecting the contrast medium (water soluble or lipiodol ultrafluid) (Fig. 77).

The contrast medium is slowly injected under low pressure. Injection stops as soon as resistance is encountered or when the patient indicates a full feeling which she can often locate in one part of the breast. The needle is then with-

Fig. 76

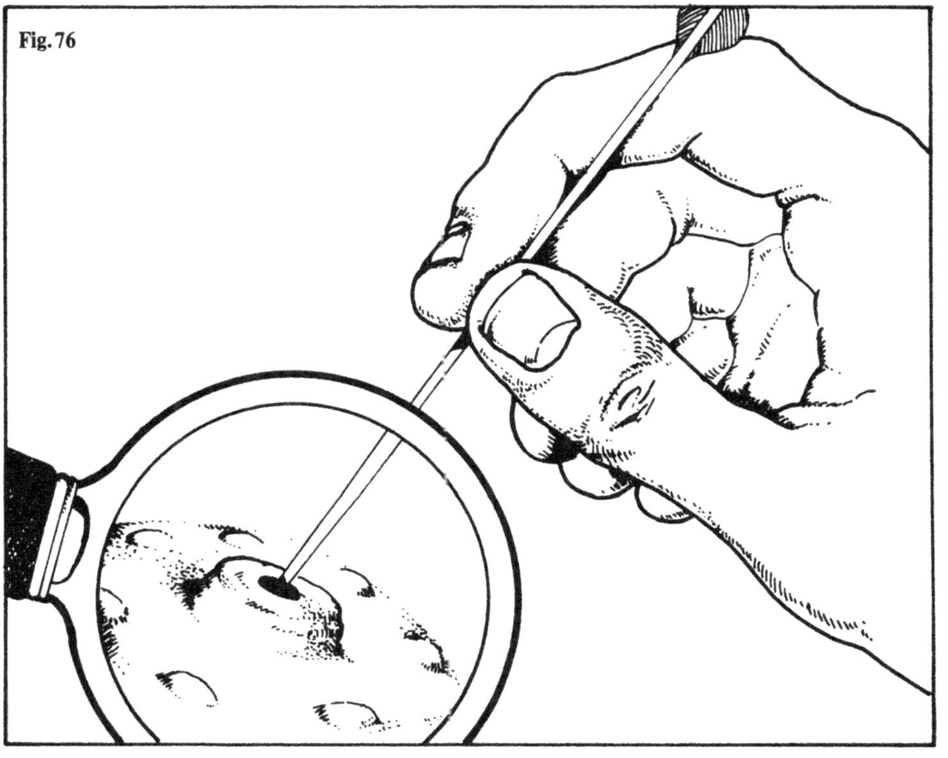

Figs. 75–77. Galactography technique:
1. Nipple compression, which may be preceded by overall breast compression, forces a droplet from one of the duct openings (the fluid may be spread on a slide for cytologic examination) (Fig. 75).
2. Gentle dilation. This is often easier if the nipple is released (Fig. 76).
3. Insertion of the soft-tipped needle. Occasionally, it is necessary to complete the catherization by slightly pulling on the nipple (Fig. 77).
4. Slow injection until resistance is felt.
5. Needle removal. Collodion or adhesive tape will seal the duct

Fig. 77

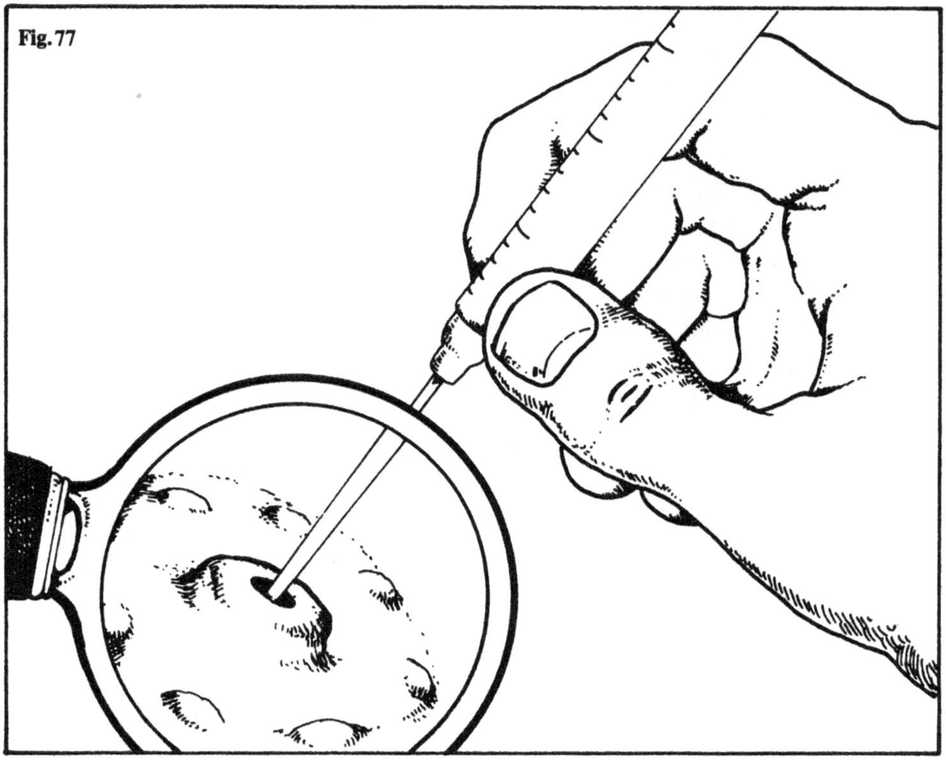

drawn while pinching the nipple. A drop of collodion or small strip of adhesive tape seals the nipple.

Three mammographic views are used: craniocaudal, latero-medial, and oblique.

At the end of the examination the adhesive tape or collodion is removed and the contrast medium evacuated as completely as possible. The patient should be warned that the discharge may change in color or quantity or may cease completely.

1.5.2.2 Interpretation

Opacification makes it possible to locate the glandular area corresponding to the affected lactiferous duct and establish its relationship to an abnormality that may appear in the mammogram. An anatomic study of the area injected will determine the degree and extent of the dilation, ductal distortion due to extrinsic factors, strictures, and intraductal vegitative processes which may or may not cause obstruction (Figs. 78–88).

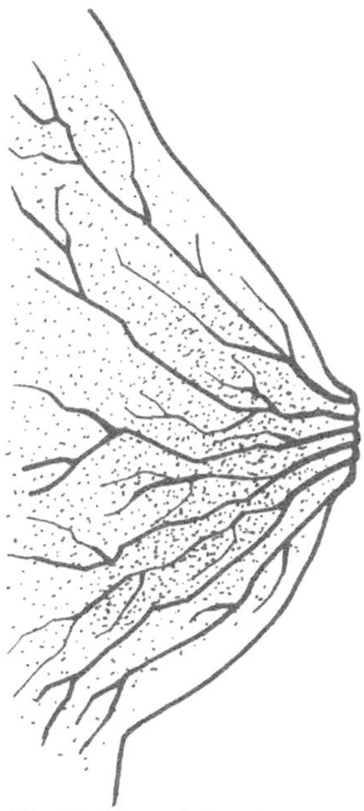

Fig. 78. Normal ductal network

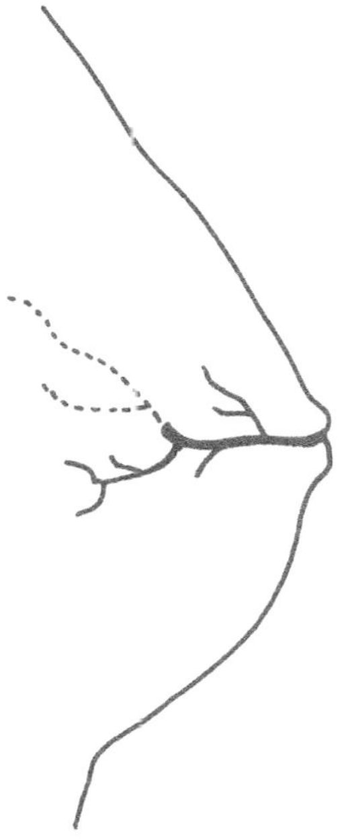

Fig. 79. Galactography: obstruction

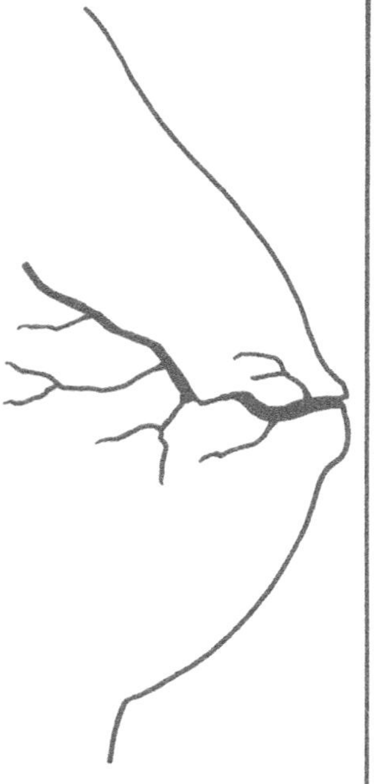

Fig. 80. Galactography: narrowing

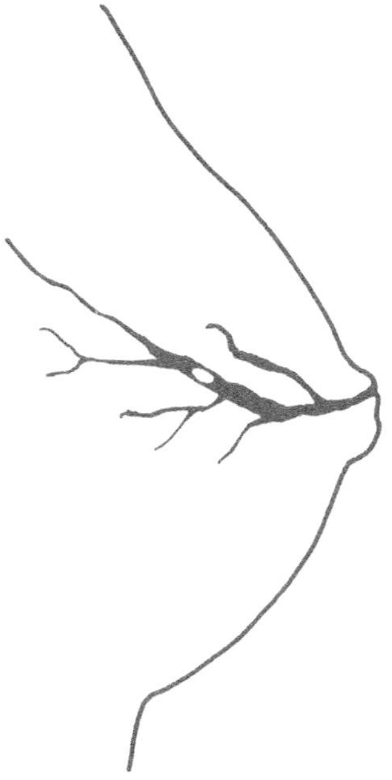

Fig. 81. Galactrography: lacuna

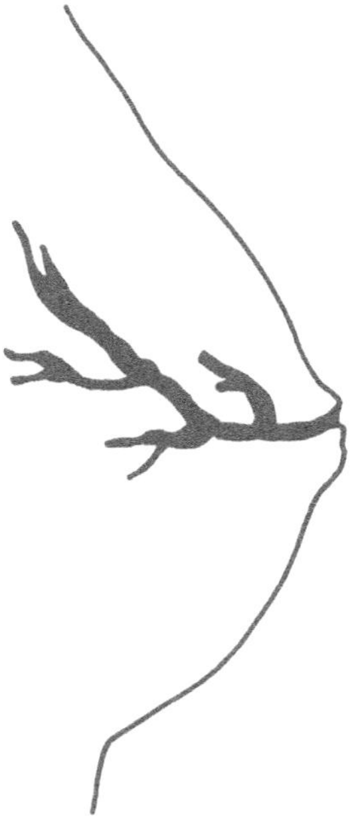

Fig. 82. Galactrography: ectasia

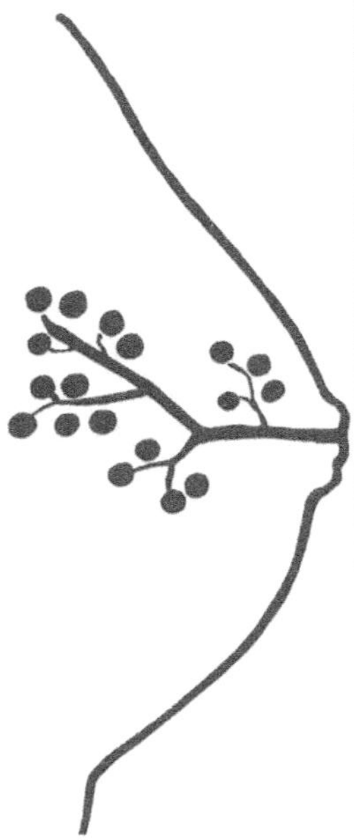

Fig. 83. Ectasia with microcysts

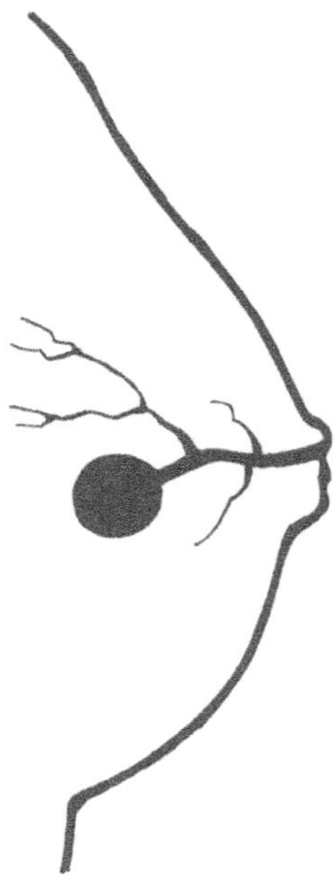

Fig. 84. Detection of a cystic cavity

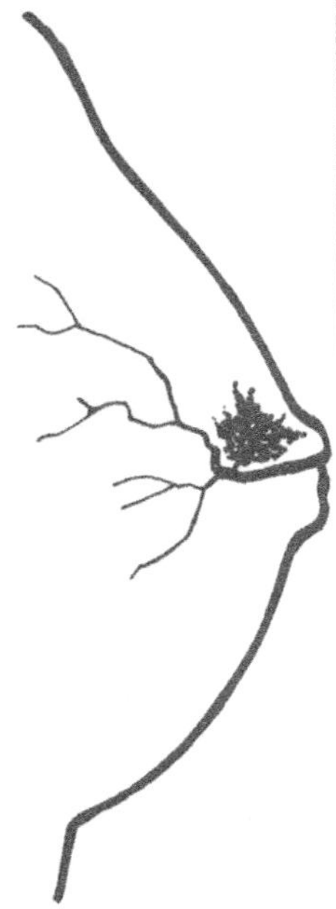

Fig. 85. Extravasation

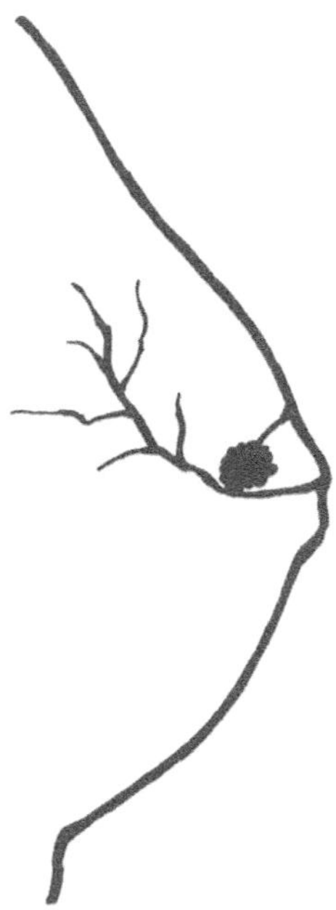

Fig. 86. Fistula

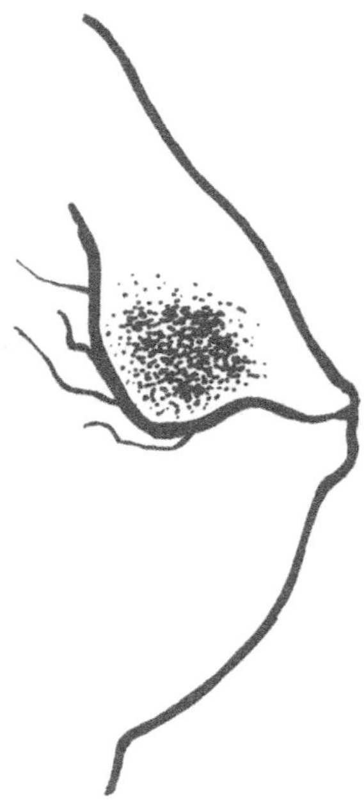

Fig. 87. Adjacent displacement

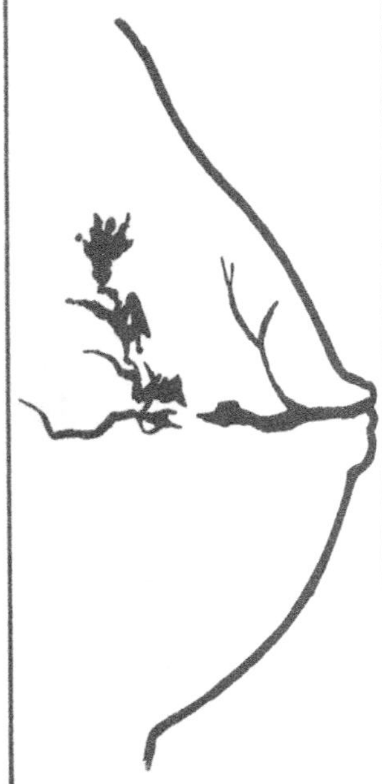

Fig. 88. Displacement with ductal change (carcinoma)

Strong Point
Monoductal lactiferous ectasia

Weak Point
Multiple ectasiae

1.5.3 Cystography

1.5.3.1 Technique (Figs. 89–92)

This is mammography after creating artificial contrast within the cyst. Air has largely replaced opaque contrast medium. Puncture-insufflation has a double role, both diagnostic: cystography (confirmed by ultrasonography) and therapeutic: air pressure within the cyst or repermeabilization of the duct generally leads to regression without relapse.

The cyst is located by palpation or ultrasound and punctured in its dependent portion with a high-gauge needle (11/10 mm). The patient may be either seated or supine. Once the fluid pushes against the plunger of the syringe, it is slowly aspirated.

Evacuation can be completed by pressing on the cyst with the other hand once the syringe is detached from the needle. It is also possible to reorient the needle, being careful not to push or pull so the needle tip will remain in the cavity. Another syringe should be filled with air, sterilized either by flame or through a sterile compress. This syringe is then very carefully attached to the needle. A volume of air equivalent or slightly greater than that of the removed fluid is injected. A sharp increase in resistance signals the end of filling. Once the needle is removed pressure is applied with gentle massage.

When there are several cysts in the same area, all the needles are left in place after puncture and all the insufflations done at the same time. This prevents one insufflated cyst from hindering the localization of the others.

Three mammographic views are used: craniocaudal, latero-medial, and oblique.

1.5.3.2 Interpretation (Figs. 93–96)

The following can be determined from the films:
- Size of the cystic cavity
- Presence of residual fluid
- Condition of the internal wall: look for vegetations

Strong Point
Solitary cyst

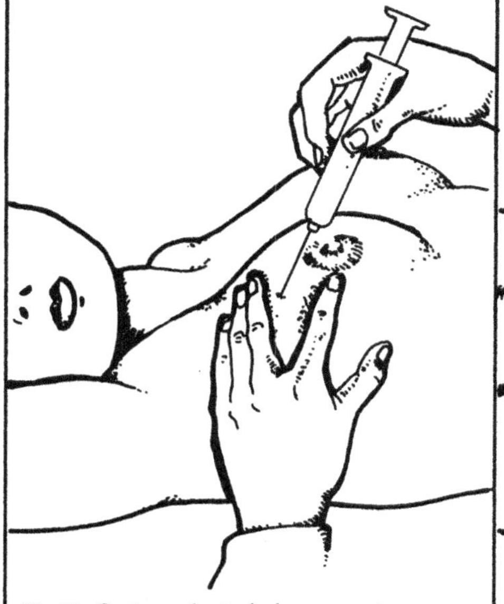

Fig. 89. Cystography technique: puncture

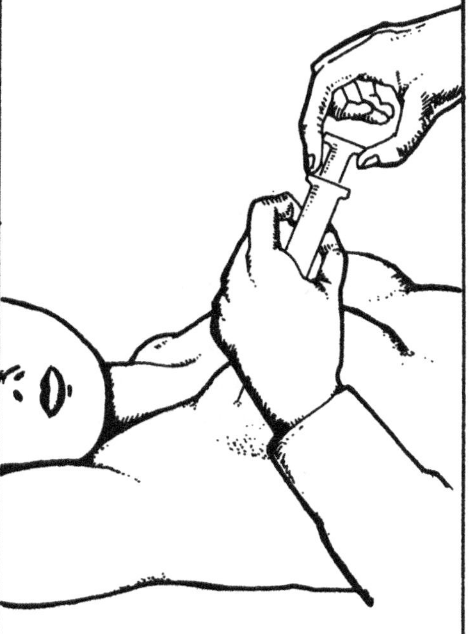

Fig. 90. Cystography technique: aspiration

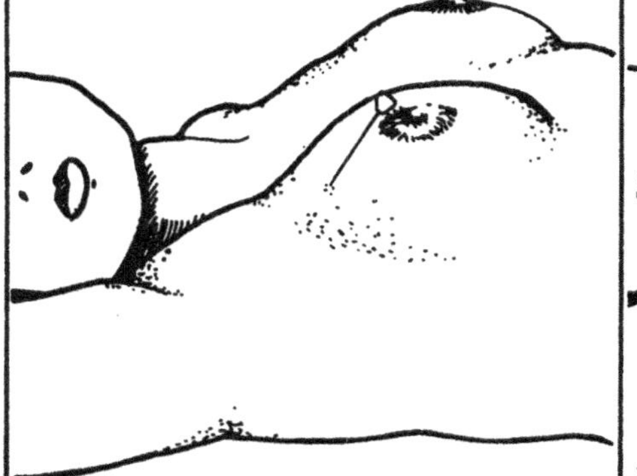

Fig. 91. Cystography technique: syringe is detached

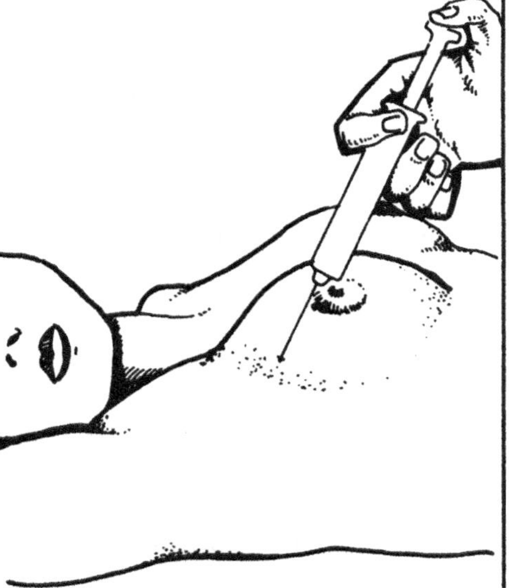

Fig. 92. Cystography technique: insufflation

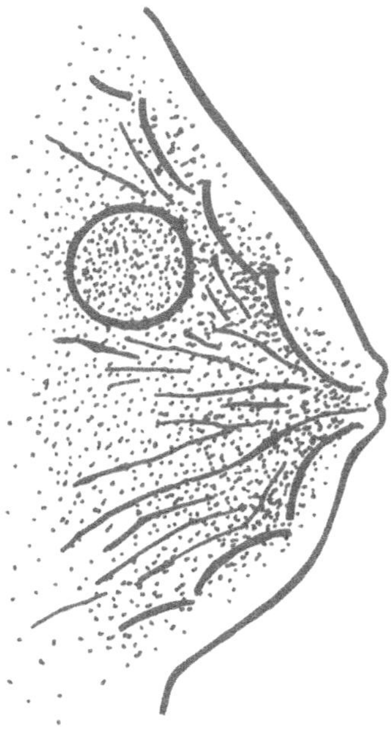

Fig. 93. Standard mammography: indistinct cyst blends in with normal opacities

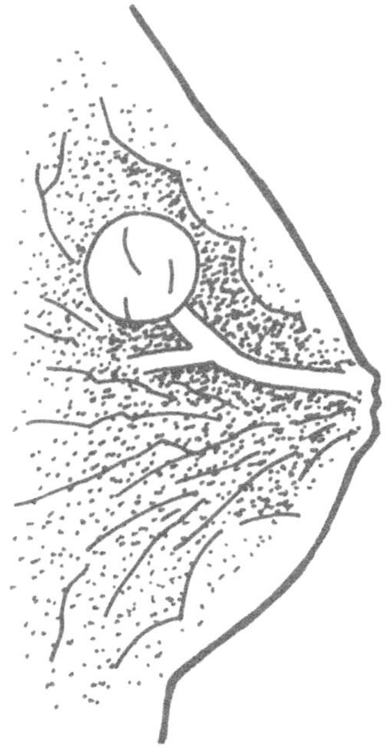

Fig. 94. Cystography: air contrast in a cyst. Air passes into a lactiferous duct

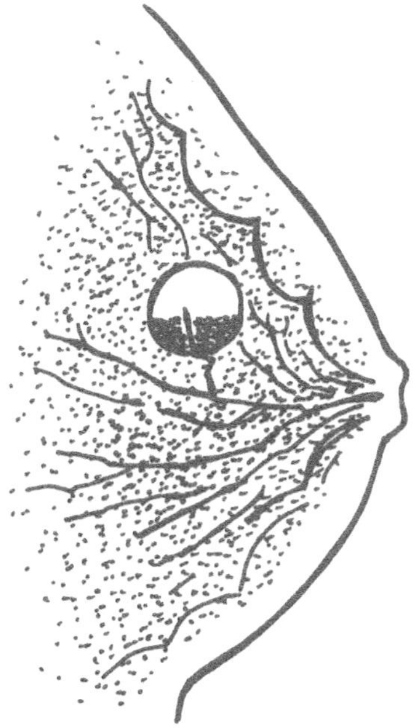

Fig. 95. Cystography: residual fluid after incomplete aspiration

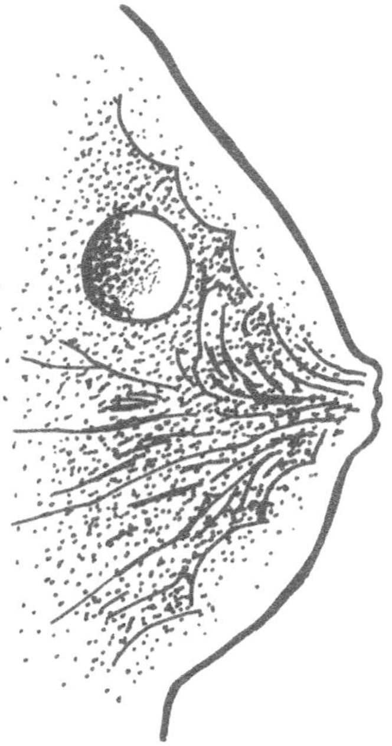

Fig. 96. Cystography: intracystic vegetations

Weak Point
Small and multiple cysts

1.5.4 Tomography

Radiographic sections of the breast may be constructed by either a mechanical or computerized process. Use of both techniques is still restricted.

1.5.4.1 Mechanical Tomography

Mechanical tomography uses the classic principle of simultaneously, similarly moved tube and film during X-ray emission. The image of each point moves at a speed that depends on the distance separating it from the film. Only that plane whose projected points move at the same speed as the film will be sharp. Kinetic blur effaces all other planes. In order to reduce radiation, several films are exposed simultaneously; a special mechanism moves them at different speeds, so that they image planes 5–10 mm apart. In this way, an entire breast can be studied with a single scan.

This type of tomography is good for analyzing images of complex elements, particularly the convergence of different bands.

1.5.4.2 Computed Tomography

Computed tomography (scanner) studies the plane scanned by a narrow beam. The intensity of the beam exiting the organ is measured point by point. There are sufficient counter-sections for the computer to reconstruct an image of the explored plane. Since images are stored in the computer, the radiologist can choose to vary individual elements of the overall image at will. The sensitivity of the technique is such that highly vascularized regions can be demonstrated by intravenous injection of contrast medium.

A special stand for use with the breast was developed and tested in the United States but has not as yet been mass produced. Whole body scanners are, thus, being used for breast examination. This reduces efficiency and increases the amount of radiation to the breast. It is especially used in the case of breast cancer.

Strong Point
Fine analysis

Weak Point
As a complementary examination

1.6 Cytodiagnosis

1.6.1 Needle Biopsy

1.6.1.1 Principles

A high-gauge needle is used to puncture a palpable lesion. Cells are then aspirated and spread on a slide for study by the pathologist. This is a highly valuable technique since it is easily performed, virtually atraumatic, and rich in information. It is important, however, to know its limits, weaknesses, and sources of error.

The aspirated cells must come directly from the lesion. The only way of being certain is if it is a palpable mass. Naturally, a lesion detected only by mammography or ultrasonography must be spatially located. In the former case, the lesion may be located with the help of a metallic grid used in place of the compression plate and held in place during puncture. In the latter case, the A sonographic curve is used to guide the needle which can be passed through a specially designed transducer (that can be sterilized). There is some risk of error with these nonmanual methods of localization. This diminishes the value of a negative result of needle biopsy performed under these conditions.

- Cells must be correctly spread.
- The biopsy must arrive at the laboratory in good condition.
- The pathologist must be trained in the particular problems of the breast. He must be informed of the clinical findings helping him to envisage each specific case. He must also be at complete liberty to indicate when a biopsy is not technically satisfactory or when he is unable to offer a clear diagnosis.

1.6.1.2 Biopsy Material

A high-gauge needle (0.8 mm), 20-ml syringe, slides, and fixative are necessary. The fixative can be either an alcohol-ether mixture into which the slide is placed or in spray form. The pathologist must be consulted concerning the choice of fixative which depends on the coloration technique to be used: Papanicolaou or May-Grunwald Giemsa.

1.6.1.3 Biopsy Technique (Figs. 97–100)

The patient is either seated or supine. The physician holds the syringe with one hand and locates and immobilizes the lump with the other. Local anesthesia, even according to the patients, is unnecessary. An alcohol base disinfectant is

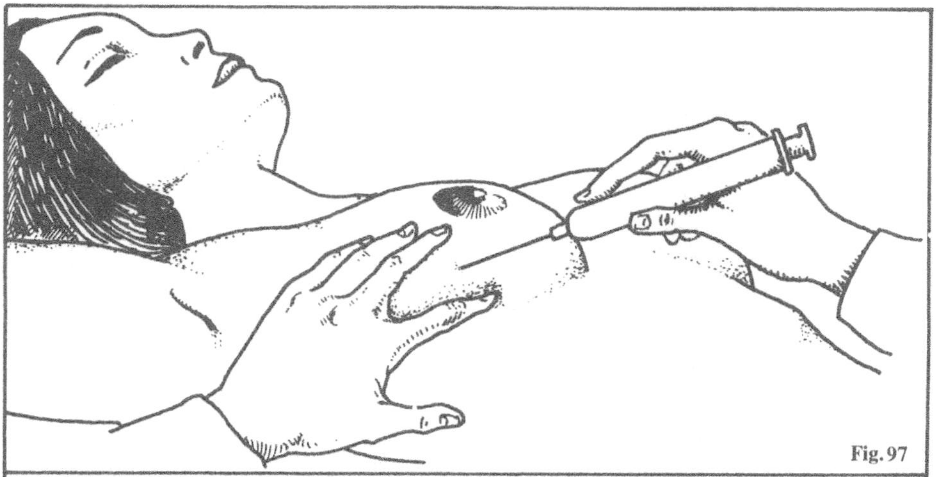

Fig. 97

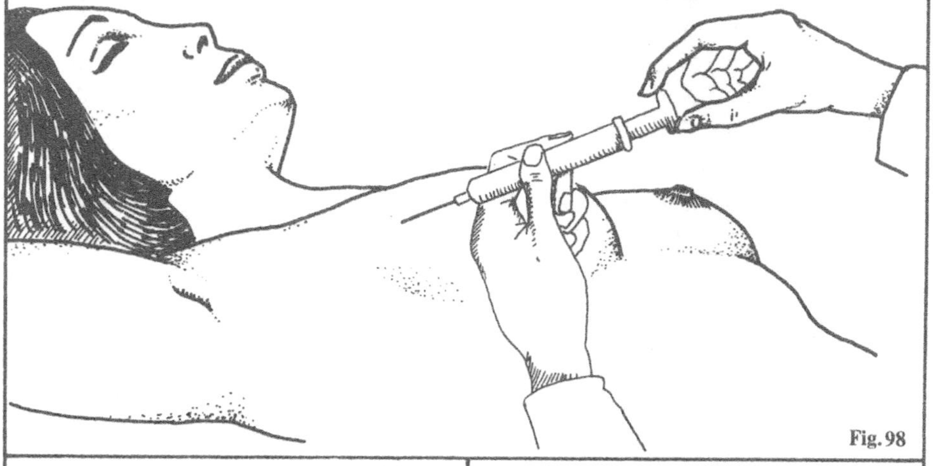

Fig. 98

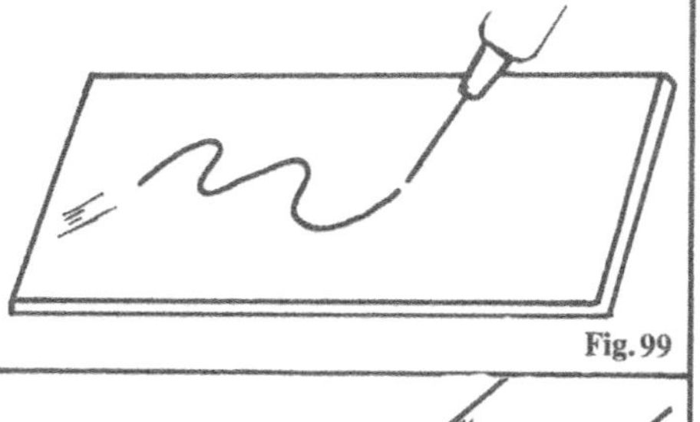

Fig. 99

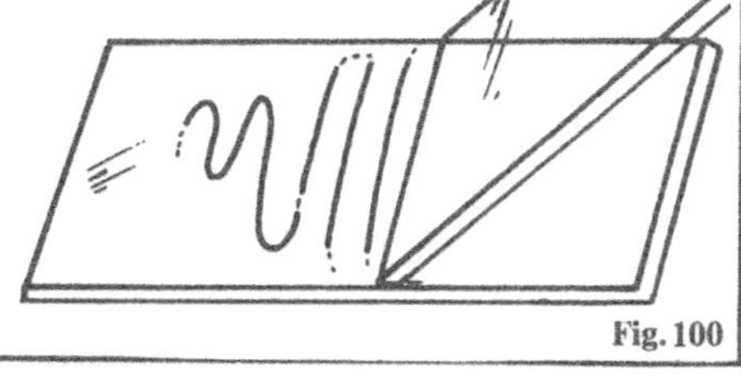

Fig. 100

Figs. 97–100. Needle biopsy technique

Fig. 97. Puncture

Fig. 98. Aspiration

Fig. 99, 100. Fluid is spread with a needle point or another slide used for local disinfection. As soon as the needle tip penetrates the tumor, the plunger of the syrine is pulled sharply but very slowly released. The needle is moved within the lesion several times with several aspirations each time. The entire aspirate remains in the needle and nothing enters the syringe. When the needle is withdrawn, an assistant or the patient herself applies firm, extended compression to the puncture site. The slide must be prepared immediately. The syringe is detached from the needle, filled with air, and reattached. A drop of the aspirate is deposited at one end of the slide by gently pushing on the plunger. The aspirate should be spread as evenly as possible using zig-zag movements of the needle. No backward movement is made in order not to disrupt the cells.

The slide is then immediately fixed. At least two slides should be prepared, one of which, according to some pathologists, should dry without fixative.

1.6.2 Cytodiagnosis of a Discharge

With spontaneous or induced unilateral discharge, a sample should be spread on a slide and fixed. Cytologic examination can prove quite valuable since adenomatous or cancerous cells may be detected.

1.6.3 Cytodiagnosis of Cystic Fluid

Once centrifuged and filtered (micropore) this fluid can undergo cytologic study. In practice it is disappointing and only rarely yields results of any real practical consequence. (Some lab series include hormonal analysis of these fluids.)

Strong Points
- Diagnosis of a well-localized lesion
- Study of a discharge

Weak Point
- Risk of false negatives

1.7 Thermography

Thermography is the study of thermal phenomena that accompany the *life* of normal and pathologic tissues. This method finds its originality in the functional nature of the information it provides as opposed to other methods of breast examination which are all morphologic and applicable to the cadaver or surgical specimen.

Only a short time ago, the supporters of telethermography (measure of infrared emitted by the skin) were strongly opposed to those of contact thermography (measure of temperature using liquid crystals). Today, each one of these methods is recognized as having its strong points and its weaknesses. Similar performances and use of a common set of signs can be achieved if both are applied with the same care and thoroughness.

1.7.1 Principles of Thermography

1.7.1.1 Physiopathologic Findings

The breast is a relatively homogeneous organ. Its functional portion consists of 15–20 lactiferous units each subject to the same endocrine effects. The metabolism, and consequently thermogenesis, of each of these elements has no appreciable difference under normal conditions. If there is a rise in thermogenesis in one or several of these units compared with the others, it makes sense that there has been a change in metabolism, or inflammation, or in any case a pathologic phenomenon. If a bilateral and overall increase in temperature of the breasts is

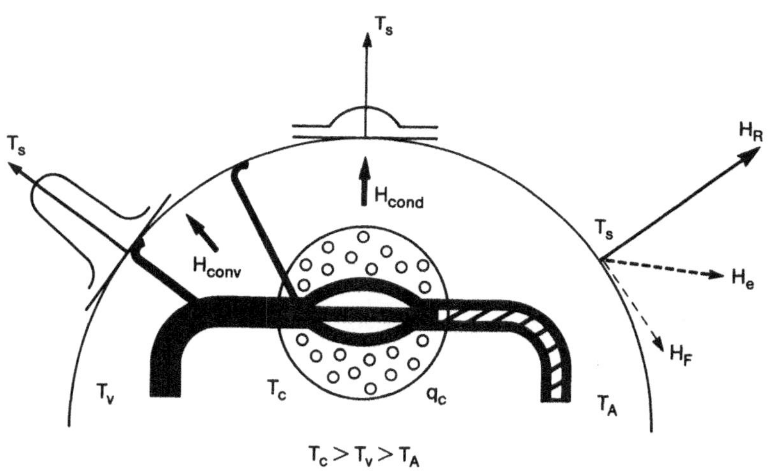

Fig. 101. Diagram of different means of caloric transfer determining skin temperature (Johansson 1976). H_F, heat loss by convection and conduction; H_e, heat loss by evaporation; H_R, heat loss by infrared rays; H_{COND}, heat transfer by conduction (tissular); H_{CONV}, heat transfer by convection (venous circulation); T_A, temperature of arterial blood; T_V, temperature of venous blood; T_C, intratumoral temperature; q_C, heat produced by tumoral cellular metabolism; T_S, temperature of the skin surface

detected, increased endocrine activity causing increased metabolism should be suspected.

In order to establish a link between deep thermogenesis and thermographic findings it is necessary to review the different processes involved.

Heat Transfer (Fig. 101)

This occurs either by conduction or convection.

- Conduction is thermal transmission by degree. Thus, the transmitted energy is proportional to the temperature gradient. It also varies with a characteristic property of the medium: its thermal conductivity. For example, the relative conductivity of different tissues, in decreasing order, has been determined experimentally: glandular tissue, fibrous tissue, and adipose tissue.
- Convection is primarily effected by blood circulation. Venous blood is warmed in areas of high metabolic activity and cooled, either in the skin or in colder areas.

Cutaneous Temperature

The thermal level of the skin depends on many factors which defy analysis: ambient temperature, air currents, hygrometry, contact and pressure on the skin, emotion, age, ect. Even after the cooling of an uncovered area removes all causes of extrinsic heating, skin temperature is not homogeneous.

- Regions closer to areas of high metabolism are warmer (by conduction).
- Superficial veins are characterized by their hyperthermia (by convection): it is believed that a vein within 7 mm of the skin provides a recognizible thermal trace.
- Calorie loss for each area, which affects its temperature, depends on the surface features (a raised zone is cooled more easily than a depressed zone).

A cutaneous thermal map is thus the result of many different factors. It would be impossible to measure precisely the temperature of one particular spot. The elements involved in creating such a temperature are too numerous and too complex. However, a measure of relative temperature (compared with the surrounding zone, the opposite side, or an anatomic reference point) is a valuable source of information providing all sources of error are systematically investigated and eliminated.

Cutaneous Heat Loss

Calories may be lost in four ways:

- Conduction through contact with clothes. This is what occurs in contact thermography but not telethermography.

- Convection due to air circulation may cause a relatively large loss. Thus, when the room is ventilated, air flow around the patient must be symmetric and homogeneous.
- Evaporation has only slight thermal effect under normal temperature and humidity conditions of the examining room.
- It is caloric loss through irradiation that is used in telethermography. This represents a major part of heat loss and can be measured directly without contact. Maximum energy is emitted in the infrared range.

1.7.1.2 Clinical Findings

In order to interpret the thermogram, it is necessary to understand the chain of events explaining how an abnormality within an organ modifies cutaneous thermal emission. A pathologic process may cause variations in thermogenesis, heat transfer, and heat loss. Several of these processes can occur simultaneously and be modified in the same or an opposing manner.

Pathologic Changes in Thermogenesis

Inflammation and growing tumors are accompanied by increased local metabolism and consequently increased heat production. It has been shown that the hyperthermia of a lesion less than 5 cm from the skin can be demonstrated by thermography. However, the lesion must be sufficiently large and warm.

Real decrease in local metabolism may occur with ischemia. An apparant decrease may be seen where there is no (cyst) or weak (lipoma) metabolic activity.

Pathologic Changes in Heat Transfer

Conduction (transfer by degree) varies with the nature of the tissue. For example, the conductance of cancerous tissue lies somewhere between that of normal glandular and fibrous tissue. Pathologic variations in heat transfer are mainly due to changes in convection. Heat transfer increases with:
- Hypervascularization surrounding a tumoral process
- Vascular dilation with inflammation
- Pathologic vascular dilation
- Collateral blood supply

and decreases with:
- Thrombosis
- Vascular spasm and stenosis

Pathologic Changes in Heat Loss

Measuring skin temperature by recording infrared emission is possible since cutaneous emission is practically constant. Variations may occur with superficial lesions: eczema, ulcerated carcinoma, etc. The temperature measured by the camera is lower than the acutal temperature. Results by contact thermography are no better since this technique needs relatively flat, smooth surfaces.

1.7.2 Physical Principles and Materials

Having established the diagnostic benefit in measuring skin temperature, we will now discuss the different practical methods. In practice, punctual or multipunctual measurements are useless. Thermography, represented by a colored image, measures all the points in a given zone.

Remember the basic physical principles making it possible to use the images of the two main techniques: contact thermography and infrared telethermography. We will only just mention microwave thermography. Theoretically, this is an enticing method since it measures the propagation of waves within tissues. Thus, it is only slightly subject to the problems of conductivity and some experiments have demonstrated its superiority. Unfortunately, it is based on the measure of very weak energies and the time needed for image construction is still too long for widespread use.

1.7.2.1 Physical Principles of Contact Thermography

Contact thermography makes use of very special physical properties of certain cholesterol substances. These substances do not have one melting point but two specific temperatures between which they take on the physical characteristics of crystals while still liquid and thus their name.

In the temperature range corresponding to this particular state, they take on a special molecular arrangement, giving them an extraordinary optical activity with the following property: the wavelength, in other words color of the reflected light, depends on the incident angle and especially the temperature. Coldest to hottest, in that order, are represented by the following colors: red, orange, yellow, green, blue, violet. It is important to note that temperature intervals are not equal for all colors. In other words it is a thermometer with unequal graduations (Fig. 102).

At first, medical use of liquid crystals was severely limited by the difficulty in applying the technique. The patient had to be painted with a layer of black paint followed by a layer of liquid crystals. Cleaning up afterwards was long and unpleasant.

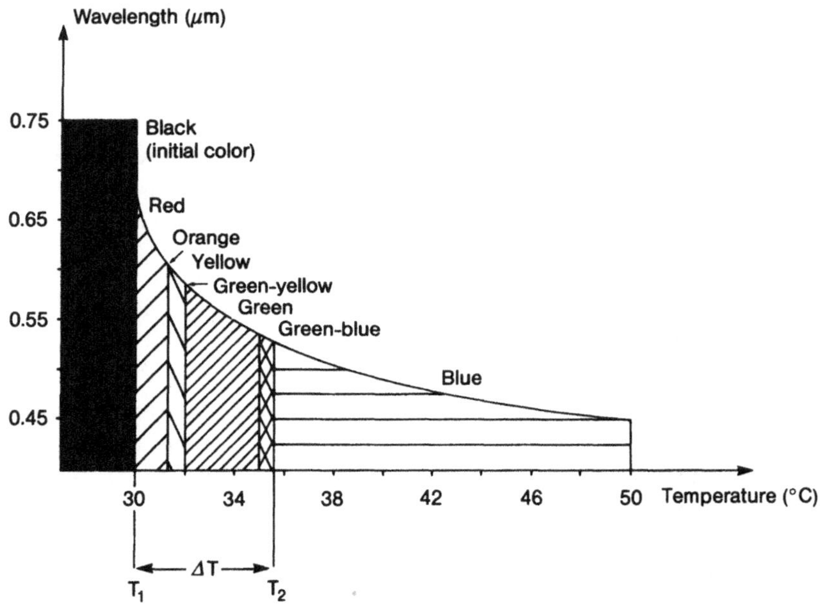

Fig. 102. Temperature intervals for contact thermography

It was not until sheets of plastic material permanently impregnated with liquid crystals on a black background were developed that use of thermography became widespread. This made it possible, by simple contact, to produce instantaneously the thermogram of an entire relatively flat area. These sheets are reusable and thus economically advantageous.

Additional advances have improved the results of contact thermography:

1. Microencapsulation of the crystals eliminates variations in the temperature-color relationship which tend to occur with aging of the substance.

2. Complex mixtures of cholesterol salts increase the range of colors which enrich and refine the thermographic image. Special mixtures have even made it possible to equalize the intervals in the temperature scale corresponding to successive colors. This means that passage from one color to the next always corresponds to the same temperature difference; for example, 0.7°C. This makes reading the thermogram considerably easier.

3. Use of an elastic base for the crystals made it possible to develop large inflatable "cushions" with a much greater active surface than conventional sheets. A thermogram of both breasts can be obtained on one single view, making detection and comparisons much easier than with the usual partial views. There are still some remaining technical problems; in particular, differences in the response of the crystals from one side to the other depending on distortion of the base.

1.7.2.2 Physical Principles of Telethermography

Since infrared emission represents a major portion of the calorie loss in humans, it was logical to consider the possibility of a quantitative and/or qualitative link between them. The problem was to determine if one could measure skin temperature at a distance using only its infrared emission.

The answer is yes, given certain factors:

Skin Temperature and Infrared Emission

All bodies emit irradiation as soon as their temperature rises above absolute zero: −273.16°C. The intensity and frequency of the irradiation are dependent on two factors: the temperature and radiant power of the body in question.

The temperature determines the emission spectrum. Planck's equation is used to calculate (for a black body) the energy emitted for a given wavelength at a given temperature. The emitted energy versus wavelength curve shows a maximum value for each wavelength. According to Wien's law, this value = 2897.76/T. (T = absolute temperature in degrees Kelvin, expressed in microns). Consequently, when the temperature rises, the wavelength corresponding to the maximum emission decreases (Fig. 103).

Radiant power is a characteristic of all surfaces. It depends on the nature of the surface and determines the percentage of irradiation emitted compared with the black body considered to be the "perfect radiator."

This radiant power varies with temperature, in other words, with the frequency emitted. Fortunately, radiant power of the skin, within an acceptable wavelength range (3–15 µm), is very close to one. Thus skin acts as an almost perfect black body as demonstrated by Henry.

Techniques for Measuring Infrared Irradiation

Different procedures have been used to produce thermograms.

- Either simultaneous recording of the entire surface to be studied. Good resolution, however, is difficult to obtain due to the weak energy of the emission. Thus, we will only mention phosphorography and evaporography. Infrared photography records irradiation from an outside source reflected off the skin.
- Or point by point recording and measurement with a scanning device. The resulting image appears on an oscilloscope and can be printed.

This point measurement of the infrared emission can be total, meaning all wavelengths are included, or selective, measuring only a narrow band of the infrared emission spectrum.

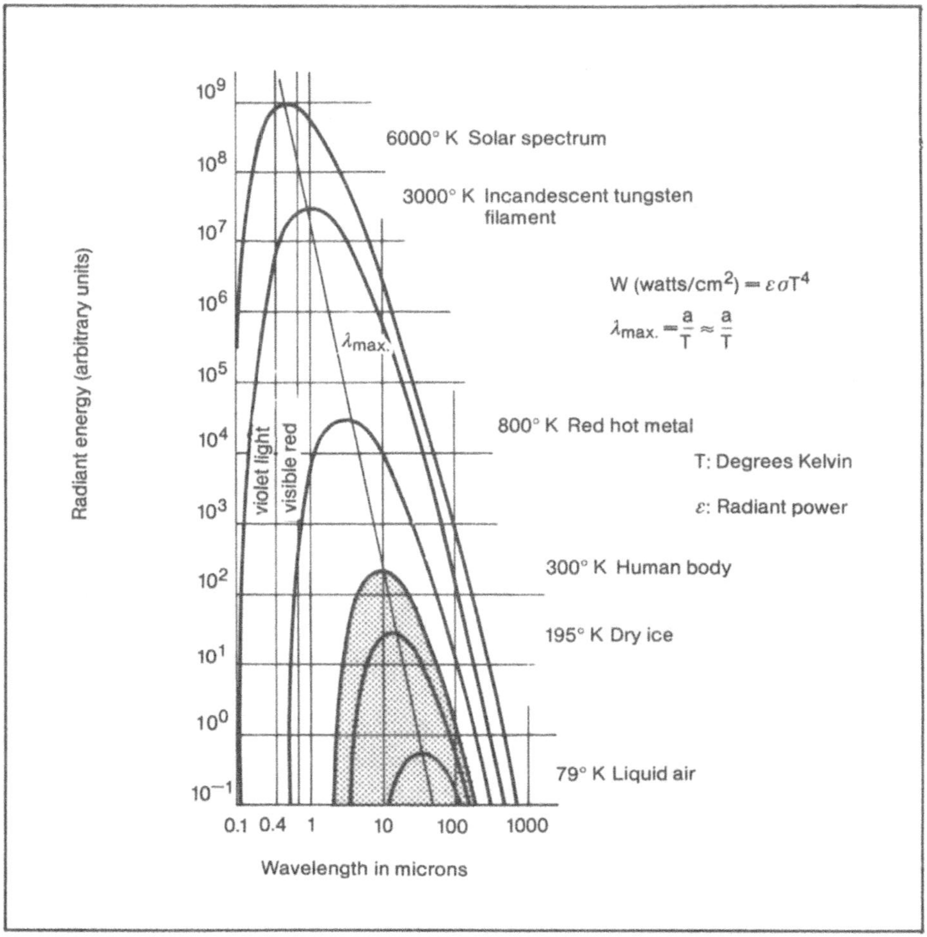

Fig. 103. Radiation emission by a black body according to temperature (Barnes 1967)

Barnes' M-1 (United States), one of the first operational units, contained a Wheatstone bridge made of a bolometric thermistor or semiconductor whose resistance varies with temperature. All of the infrared irradiation emitted combined to alter the temperature of the thermistor, thus destabilizing the bridge, producing a measurable current.

Present-day thermographs (Fig. 104) are based on the principle of seletively measuring a narrow band of infrared frequency. They use an antimonium of indium photoconductor whose sensitivity is maximum at a frequency of 5 µm and practically zero beginning with 6 µm. The beam first passes through a germanium filter which absorbs visible and near infrared (less than 2 µm) rays (Fig. 105).

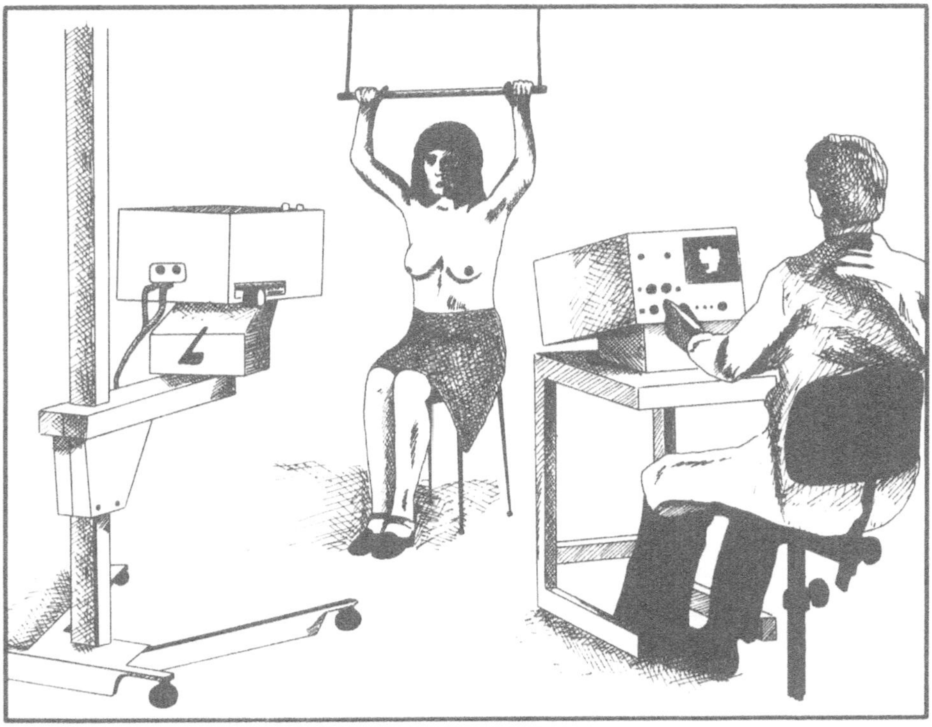

Fig. 104. Thermographic examination of the breasts (Philips thermograph)

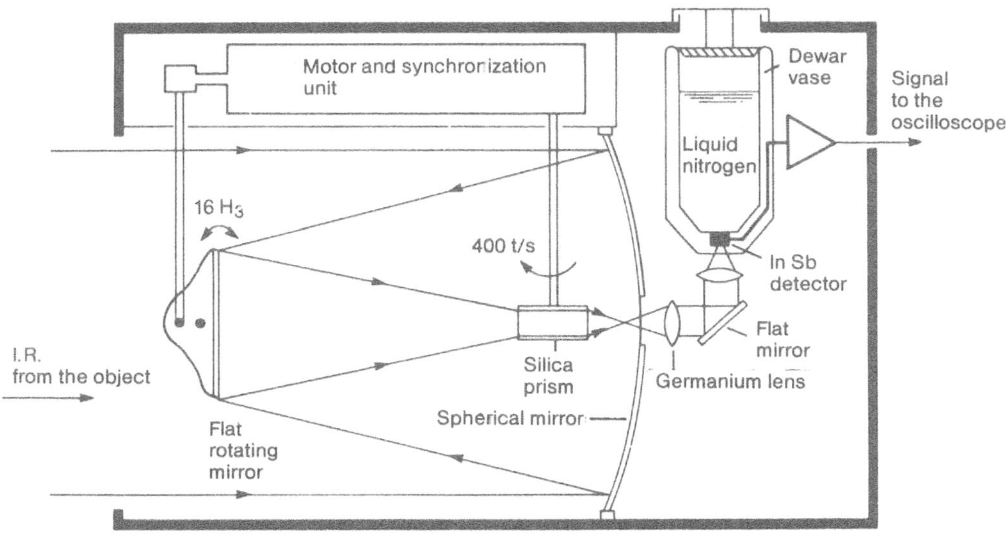

Fig. 105. Simplified diagram of a telethermographic camera (thermovision Aga)

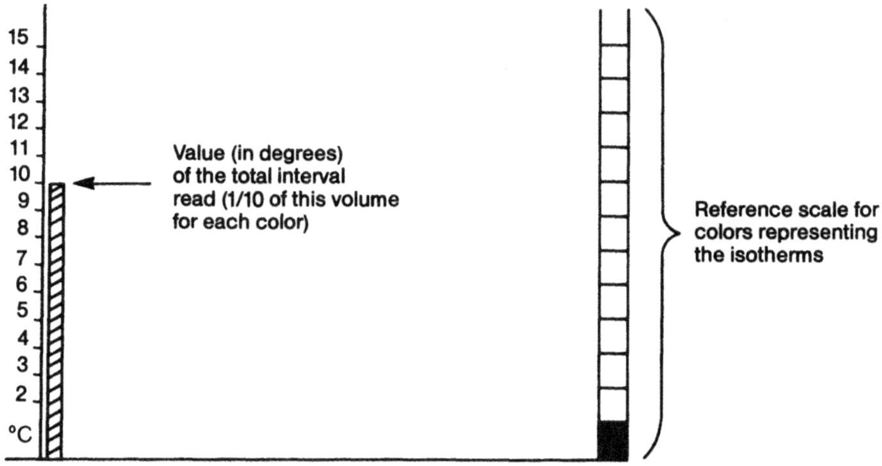

Fig. 106. Color thermogram

Consequently, the measurement is made in a band containing only 2% of the total energy emitted. Other photoconductors can also be used: tellurium of cadmium, and mercury, which picks up 35% of the emitted energy. For temperatures close to 300°K (27°C), percentage variations of emission in the 5- to 6-μm band are equivalent to the change in absolute temperature to the tenth power. For the total infrared band, however, this is only raised to the fourth power. With antimonium of indium, then, there is a considerable increase in the sensitivity to temperature changes and thus an increase in contrast of the signals.

A point detector analyzes the image with double scanning by a system of rotating mirrors. The design engineer must compromise in order to take into account two opposing parameters: total scanning speed, which determines the number of images per second, and the sharpness of the thermogram, which depends on the number of points measured. In 1/16 of a second, 10000 points can be recorded (100 lines, 100 points per line); in ½ of a second the number increases to 42000 points (160 lines, 260 points per line).

Practical Use of Infrared Measurement

The electric signal can be projected on a screen which in turn can be photographed using standard or instantaneously developed film. For a direct image, the warmer the point, the whiter its image or vice versa (the opposite mode is easier to read); with certain controls, the examiner can choose the temperatures to be measured; in other words, the temperature interval producing shades of gray that form the image. In direct mode, all points whose temperature is lower

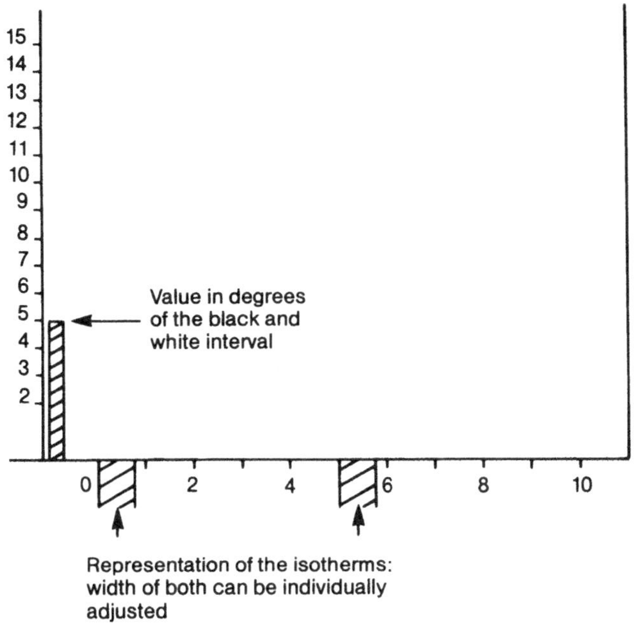

Fig. 107. Black and white thermogram

than this interval will appear black and all points of higher temperature will be white.

It is possible to regulate not only the heat level of the interval but also its width; for example: from 28° to 35°C or from 30° to 32°C. This will vary the contrast (Fig. 106).

All points whose temperatures fall between two values chosen at will can appear as either white or black on the thermogram. Two isothermic intervals can be displayed simultaneously so the temperature difference between two points may be read instantly (Fig. 107).

The color thermogram represents the most elaborate use of isotherms. All points whose temperatures are within the selected interval will appear in color on the same image. Each color (seven to ten depending on the unit) corresponds to an isotherm and, thus, to a temperature. The color order from coldest to warmest is arbitrarily determined by the designer but may be reversed by the examiner.

Color thermograms can be produced in two ways:

- A black and white oscilloscope is photographed with color film while white isotherms are successively shown. A rotating disk places a filter of the corresponding color in front of the lens. This device requires a fairly long exposure time.
- A color oscilloscope directly projects the image, whose isotherms are electrically analyzed simultaneously.

Electronics offers another possiblity: the thermal profile. A horizontal scanning line is replaced by a temperature curve. This technique is rarely used in practice.

With digitalization of the signal a new generation of thermographs has developed with the possibility of freezing the color image on the screen.

This image can then be studied at a later time. In addition, the outline of a rectangular zone, whose location and dimensions are selected by the examiner, can be projected on the screen. The unit instantly displays the thermal index, which is the average temperature of the selected area. If applicable to breast examination, this device would be of great benefit. Unfortunately, a rectangular surface can rarely be adapted to a breast image.

1.7.3 Thermographic Techniques

Conditions of the examination should be chosen in order to eliminate, or at least reduce, causes of error and to decrease basal heat emission in order to achieve the greatest contrast possible at significant heat emission. Inflammation, certain local treatments, and the menstrual cycle (avoid the second half) may all affect the technique. The patient, disrobed from the waist up and with nothing touching the breasts, should sit in a temperature-controlled room (20°–22°C) for approximately 15 min prior to the examination.

In some cases important additional information can be obtained by the forced cooling test with contact as well as infrared thermography. After the initial examination ventilation is used to cool the skin rapidly. The time required for a warm spot to reappear is then determined. In principle, carcinoma is suspected with rapidly reappearing hyperthermia (1 min).

Pharmacodynamic tests based on the role of insulin and glucose in cancer metabolism have not as yet yielded convincing statistics but may not be entirely without merit.

1.7.3.1 Special Aspects of Contact Thermography

Choice of the liquid crystal sheet depends on the unit. Temperature ranges differ for a varying number of colors. Generally we begin with a sheet which records down to 33°C. With strong cooling, however, it is often necessary to use a sheet with a lower range. The choice is easy since the results are instantly displayed.

When applying the sheet, it is important to locate and center the nipple.

The patient raises her arms and two views are taken of each breast:

- A coronal view, nipple at the center of the sheet
- A lateral profile view, nipple near the anterior edge of the sheet

Other views may be necessary depending on the patient's build or in the case of a previously detected abnormality.

The examination should be performed rapidly since contact with the sheets may increase skin temperature. The examiner, then, should be more concerned with carrying out a high-quality examination since interpretation of the results may be done at a later date.

1.7.3.2 Special Aspects of Telethermography

There are two phases to the examination:

- A black and white image is produced by analogic conversion. This makes it possible to study the thermovascular appearance. While observing the screen, the following adjustments are made:
  Centering, the entire thorax is included
  Optical, according to the distance
  Electric, according to the skin temperature and the best range yielding the best contrast. All these adjustments should be made within a few seconds. At least one coronal film and occasionally some oblique films are then made
- A color image is produced by digital conversion. To facilitate the reading, we choose a simple value between two successive colors 0.2°C, 0.5°C, or most often 1°C. The temperature range is chosen after verifying that all areas will be covered, in other words, that there are no entirely black patches (setting too high) or white patches (setting too low).

This adjustment takes only a few seconds. With the patient's arms still raised, three images are recorded: one coronal and two oblique.

For some patients with large pendulous breasts, the examination may have to be done with the patient in the supine position for the lower quadrants.

1.7.3.3 Some Easily Avoided Pitfalls

Since skin temperature is altered, sometimes for hours, by palpation and even more so by mammography, these procedures should never precede thermography.

Needle biopsy only slightly affects the thermogram: a 4-day interval should be sufficient.

A pressed or prolonged application of the sheets in contact thermography may cancel the effect of cooling.

1.7.4 Thermographic Interpretation

Contact and infrared thermography both work differently depending on the type of symptom studied. With this in mind, it is possible to use the same basic signs for both.

1.7.4.1 Basic Signs

Superficial Vascularization

There are six vascular types (Fig. 108):
- Type A: avascular breasts
- Type B: fairly extensive, evenly distributed linear vascularization
- Dystrophic type B: same distribution but with thick traces and many coral branch and mimosa images
- Type C: localized, irregular vascularization of uneven distribution: vascular star with four or more branches, vascular circle with partial radial vascular trace
- Type D: vascular network
- Type E: spotted vascularization seen on the breasts as well as the entire thorax

The type of vascularization is only one element of interpretation. Nevertheless, each type is seen more often in given circumstances; type A, at rest, especially in elderly women; type B, during the first part of the menstrual cycle; dystrophic type B, during the second half of the cycle or with estrogen hyperactivity: type C, with carcinoma; type D, during pregnancy or lactation; and type E, in so-called neurotonic subjects.

Vascular asymmetry (different types at right and left) is a pathologic sign.

Localized Hyperthermia

This may be detected in one or more areas of variable size. It is either homogeneous or in the form of vascular images. It is particularly significant if 2°C or more than the corresponding area of the other breast. Comparison with the temperature of the xyphoid region appears to have been abandoned since it is imprecise and cannot be used in contact thermography.

Fig. 108. Breast thermovascular patterns: *Type A* "Uniform avascular." Thermal distribution is uniform. Thermovascular traces are absent or very slight. *Type B* "Linear vascular." One or several thermovascular traces are observed in one or several quadrants. *Type B+* "Dystrophic vascular." Thermovascular traces are even but longer and thicker than in type B. They may have a "coral branch" appearance. When associated with small thermal spots, they have a characteristic "mimosa branch" appearance. *Type C* "Irregular vascular." Numerous, grouped, but irregularly distributed signs of vascular hyperthermia. *Type D* "Network vascular." Thermovascular network pattern. *Type E* "Spotted avascular." Hyperthermic patches of variable size spread over the breasts and thorax (may be transitory, especially in emotional patients)

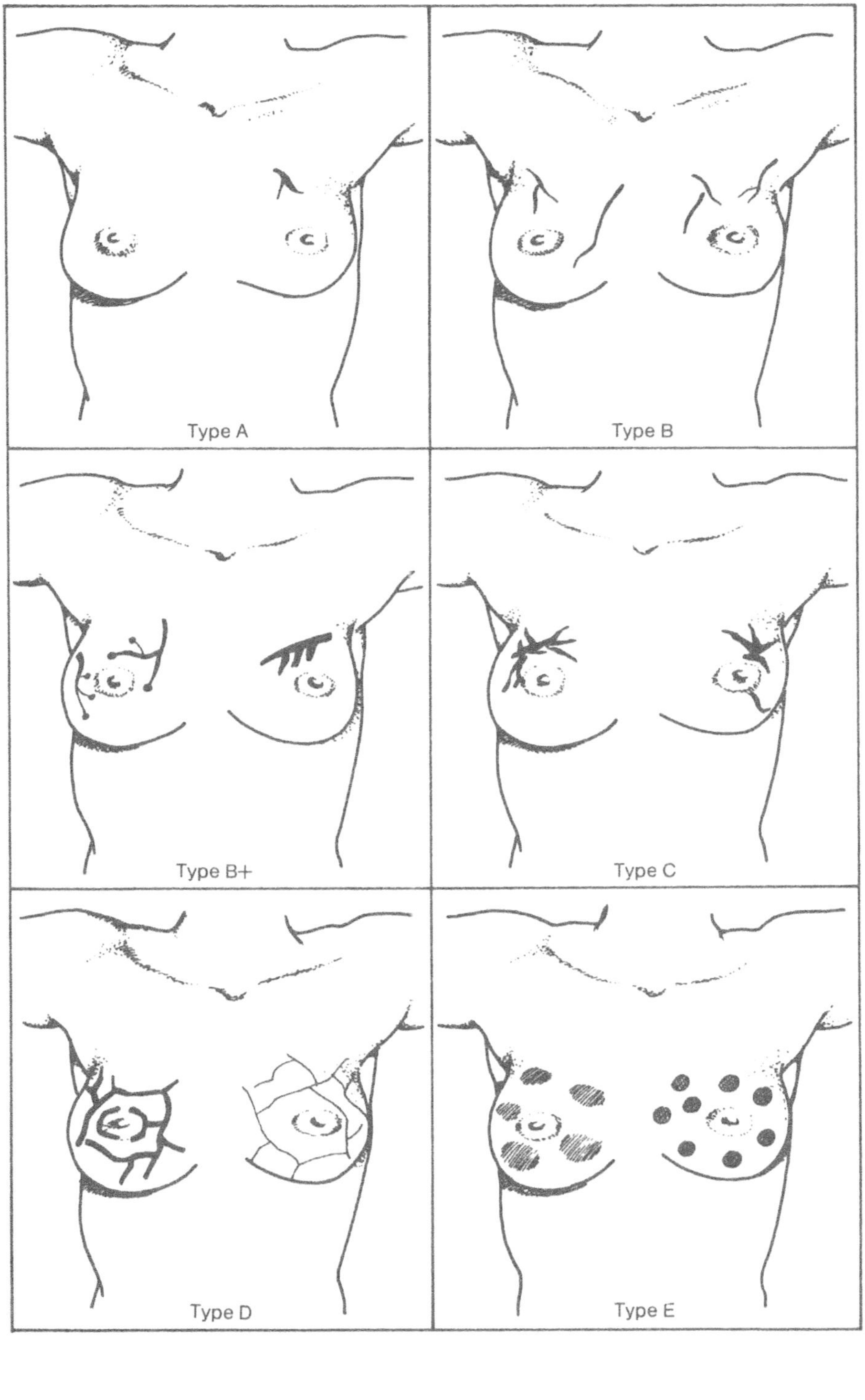
Type A
Type B
Type B+
Type C
Type D
Type E

NB. It is mostly likely due to strong cooling that the Marseille authors obtain very high thermal gradients			**Marseille** classification			**Strasbourg** classification
						Eight basic signs from a to h
Vascular anomalies	Symmetric hypervascul-arization 1	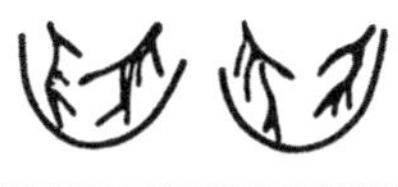	1			
	Asymmetric hypervascul-arization 2	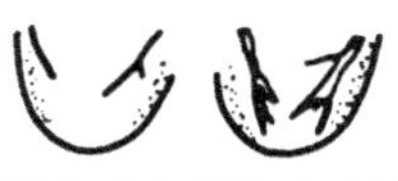		1		h) Different thermal topography between the two breasts
	Irregular hypervascul-arization 3	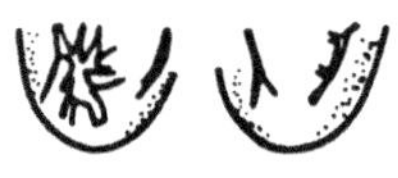			1	g) Type C vascular pattern (irregular vascular)
Hot zone	Moderate 4	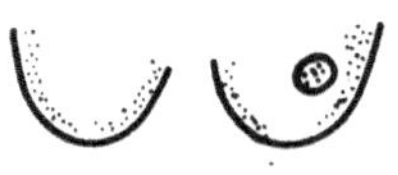	1 ≤2°			a) One hot zone. If it represents a vascular zone, it is not valid unless sign b is noted
	Average 5	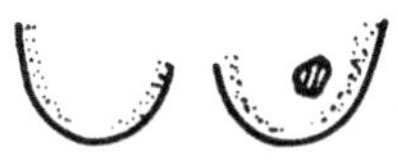		1 2.5°		a + b) More than 2°C compared with symmetric area
	High 6	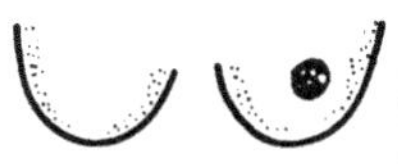			1 ≥3°	a + b + c) More than 1.5°C compared with xiphoid reference
Overall hyper-thermia of one breast	Moderate 7	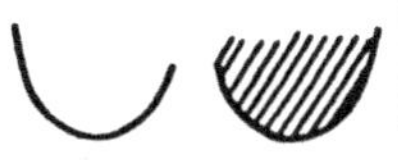		1 2°		e) More than 1.5°C compared with the other breast
	High 8	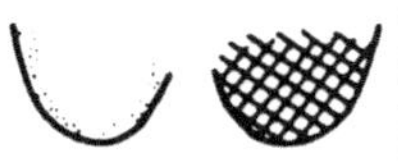			1 ≥2°	e + f) Overall temperature of the breast is higher than that of the xiphoid reference
Deter-mination of thermal contour ("edge sign")	Limited 9	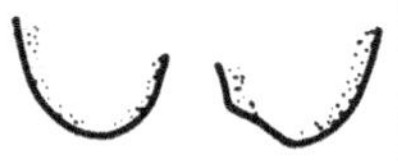		1		
	Extensive 10				1	
Thermo-clinical or thermo-radiographic correlation	Topographic correlation between hot zone and cli-nical nodule or radiograph-ic opacity 11	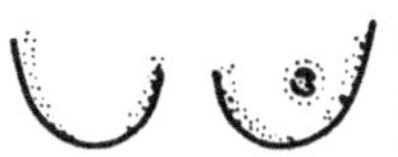				d)

Fig. 109. Pathologic signs in breast thermography (schools of Marseille and Strasbourg)

Total Hyperthermia

Total hyperthermia of one breast compared with the other is pathologic if the difference is greater than 1°C.

Concordance

Concordance between a thermographic anomaly and a clinical, radiographic or sonographic abnormality is undoubtedly a valuable element but must be considered as part of the overall clinical picture.

Distortion

Distortion of the breast's thermal contour corresponds to retraction. Even if only minor, it has usually already been detected during the clinical examination. This is not really considered a thermographic sign even if in some cases it has led to detection. Symptoms related to vascular morphology are more easily demonstrated by contact thermography. Infrared thermography is better for quantitatively determining temperature differences. Nevertheless, the different types of thermograms can be obtained by the correct use of either method.

1.7.4.2 Diagnostic Classification (Fig. 109)

In order to avoid all misunderstanding, it should be clear that thermography alone is no better able to make a diagnosis than the hands of a clock are of telling time without the face. Thermography gives a qualitative and quantitative indication of the organism's reaction without specifying to what it is due. It does, however, provide valuable information when performed in conjunction with other morphologic examinations.

All of the basic signs described above must be taken into account in order to classify the thermogram. Protocols may vary among different schools but are fundamentally the same. We usually refer to the Strasbourg classification, which is precise and takes both thermographic methods into account. Thermograms are classified from TH1 to TH5 in the same manner as Papanicolaou's cytologic classification (Table 1). We do feel, however, that the use of the adjectives applied to each class (normal, benign, questionable, suspicious, and highly suspicious) as used in the examination report is awkward, illogical, and often premature.

1.7.4.3 Prognostic Classification

When carcinoma is diagnosed, thermography can be used to establish a prognosis. Once again, we use the Strasbourg classification, which has been the

Table 1. Breast: comparison between the classifications of Marseille and Strasbourg

	Marseille (Amalric)	Strasbourg (Gros)
TH1 (normal)	Normal thermogram	No basic thermo-pathologic sign
TH2 (benign)	Abnormal thermogram: benign type	One or two signs
TH3 (doubtful)	Suspect thermogram (one sign of suspicion)	Three signs, except (a, b, e) or (a, b, g)
TH4 (malignancy is suspect)	Thermogram with one criterion of malignancy or several signs of suspicion	Four or five signs, or (a, b, e) or (a, b, g)
TH5 (malignancy is highly suspect)	Thermogram with several criteria of malignancy	Six, seven, or eight signs

Table 2. Prognostic classification of the thermogram (Strasbourg school)

Q0	No pathologic sign
Q1	One, two, or three basic pathologic signs except (a, b, e) associated
Q2	(a + b + e) or four or five signs with (a or e)
Q3	Four or five signs with (a + e)
Q4	Six, seven, or eight basic pathologic signs

object of a long-term statistical study. Thermograms are classified from Q0 (noninvasive lesion) to Q4 (carcinomatous mastitis) (Table 2).

The Marseille school uses a tumoral growth index: $I = \Delta 2/S$; $\Delta 2$ is the temperature difference between the two sides in tenths of a degree; S is the hyperthermic surface:
$S1$ = less than half the breast
$S2$ = between one-half and the entire breast
$S3$ = more than the entire breast
When I is greater than 50, tumor growth is rapid.

1.7.4.4 Interpretation and Follow-up

In the case of follow-up examinations, the radiologist must compare the current thermogram with previous films.

Whether it be a functional test (examination after hormonal treatment) or reexamination of an isolated thermographic abnormality, it is important first to test the technique on neutral areas: shoulders, cervical region. In this way, adjustments can be made to avoid errors in interpretation: for physical or physiological reasons, thermograms may differ either in total thermal level or degree of contrasts.

Strong Point
Small developing lesions

Weak Point
Lack of specificity

1.8 Invasive Examination

1.8.1 Nonsurgical Biopsy

Drill biopsy for histologic examination is a borderline invasive technique. It offers a more accurate diagnosis than needle aspiration since it provides fragments showing tissue structure. This technique is more aggressive than needle aspiration but is generally well tolerated. While there is no longer any question about the harmlessness of needle biopsy, there is some evidence that drill biopsy may activate cancer. It is also important to note that this type of biposy may lead to the formation of scar tissue, making future examinations difficult.

1.8.2 Open Biopsy

1.8.2.1 Preoperative Mammographic Localization

Different techniques have been suggested to help the surgeon operate, with sufficient precision, on radiographically detected nonpalpable lesions. Here, we describe the Lamarque technique:

- A guided needle is inserted into the lesion and its position verified by two mammograms (Fig. 110).
- The guide is withdrawn and a mixture of xylocaine and methylene blue is injected (for postoperative localization) (Fig. 111).
- A hooked wire is threaded through the needle to the lesion (Fig. 112).
- The needle is withdrawn and the wire is fastened to the skin. This wire will provide both surgical and radiographic localization (Fig. 113).

1.8.2.2 Pathologic Study

For a number of reasons, there is now some doubt concerning what not long ago was the systematic frozen section diagnosis:

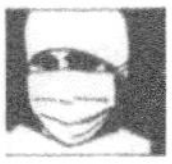

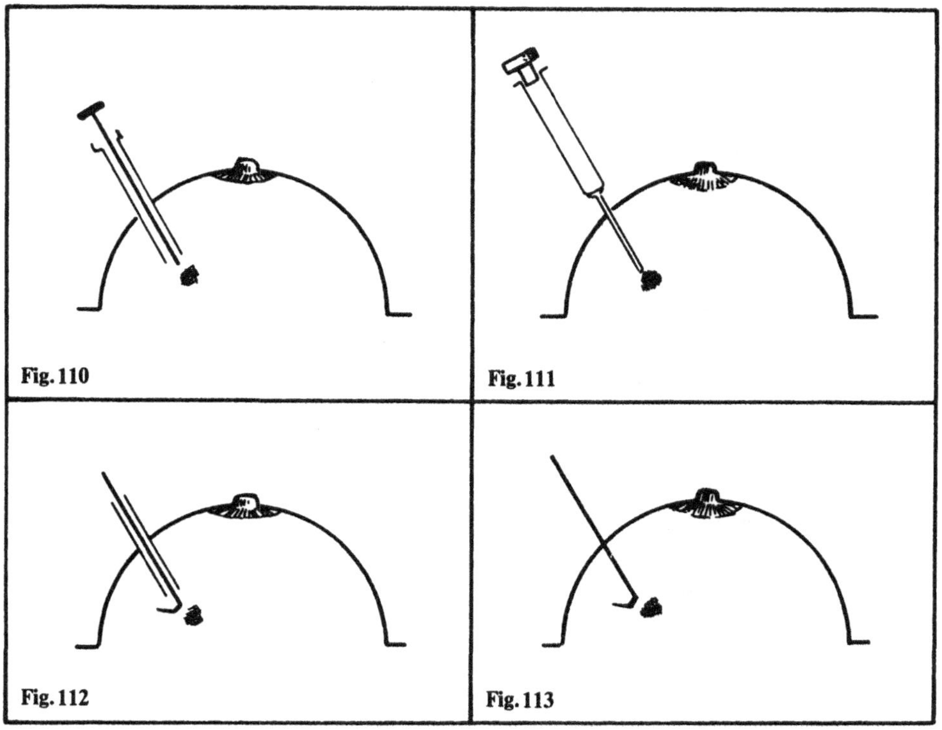

Fig. 110–113. Radiographic localization of a nonpalpable lesion. (Technique described by J. L. Lemarque 1981)

Conditions under which the pathologist must examine the slides are not the best especially since time is limited:

- The freezing technique in itself may in some cases make examination difficult
- During this surgery, a diagnosis of carcinoma and the need for what may be mutilating therapy represents a situation which is difficult for the surgeon and traumatic for the patient.

1.8.2.3 Specimen Radiography

This technique applies to biopsies of nonpalpable lesions detected by mammography. The film is taken by a mammography unit with film alone or single-layer film with a screen. If the biopsy is incomplete, the surgeon can then immediately excise additional tissue.

Strong Point

- Provides a histologic specimen

Table 3. Basic symptomatology: response of the different tissues for each type of examination

	Clinical: firmness	Trans-illumination: trans-parency	Ultra-sound: echo-genicity	Ultra-sound: beam absorp-tion	Mammo-graphy: opacity	Thermo-graphy: heat trans-mission	
Connective tissue-ductal network	=	=	=	=	=	=	Anatomic elements
"Passive" mesenchyma (fatty tissue)	–	+	–	–	–	–	
Vessels	=	–	=	=	=	++	
Nerves	=	=	=	=	=	=	
Skin	=	=	=	=	+	=	
Nipple-areolar area	+	–	=	+	+	–	
Lymph nodes	+	=	=	=	=	=	
Excess hydration	+	+	–	–	+	–	Changes in the basic tissues
Fibrosis	=	–	+	+	=	+	
Calcifications	+ (if large size)	–	+	++	++	–	
Epithelial proliferation	=	–	+	+	+	+	

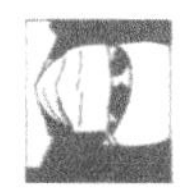

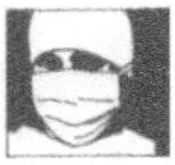

Weak Points
- Localization of nonpalpable lesions
- May cause problem scaring

1.9 Magnetic Resonance Imaging

While not yet widely used, MRI should be mentioned since it may prove valuable in breast examination. The principle can be simplified and summarized as follows:

Under the effect of a magnetic field, protons will resonate with an electromagnetic field. When the stimulus stops, the protons return to their resting state. The length of time for this return, which is variable, is measured. It gives an indication of the quantity of certain elements forming the tissue of the examined area.

Hydrogen contained in the water is thus detected and evaluated. A tomographic-type image can be produced in which neoplastic edematous infiltration can be detected.

Currently the cost and complexity of MRI equipment is discouraging.

Hopefully, future research will improve this situation.

Strong Point
- High specificity

Weak Points
- Cost
- Still being developed

2 Normal Breasts

Major anatomic variations from one woman to another and in the same woman from one time to another make the breast a unique organ: an organ-event. Rather than describe a perfect structure that does not exist, we will try to cover the processes that lead to development and changes in the breasts.

In the beginning, there was ectoderm. At birth, the nipple and a definitive number of lactiferous duct elements are already formed. The breast remains in an infantile state until prepuberty. At this time, its development signals the beginning of sex hormone activity.

Lactiferous ducts and their finger-like or alveolar endings are the specific receptors of hormone activcity. They are capable of major development and regression. The surrounding connective and fatty tissues are not unaffected by hormones but their development is less rapid. The supporting connective tissue and skin show the effects of major growth periods. Fatty tissue is affected by both the morphologic development of the breast, controlled by the sex hormones, and the women's general metabolism.

2.1 Breast Tissue and Examination Findings

The breast develops between the fascia pectoralis and its skin covering. Fifteen to 20 lactiferous ducts converge toward its anatomic center, the mammary papilla (nipple). Each duct corresponds to a lobe which itself is divided into numerous lobules. While apparently separate, the lobes are joined by several lactiferous anastomoses. Connective tissue forms fibrous bands known as Cooper's ligaments which course through the breast from the deep fascia to the dermis of the skin where they attach to Duret's crests.

2.1.1 Lactiferous-Connective Tissue Network (Fig. 114)

It is impossible to distinguish between the different histologic elements of this network by noninvasive examination except through creation of artificial radiologic contrast: air galactograms and particularly opaque galactography.

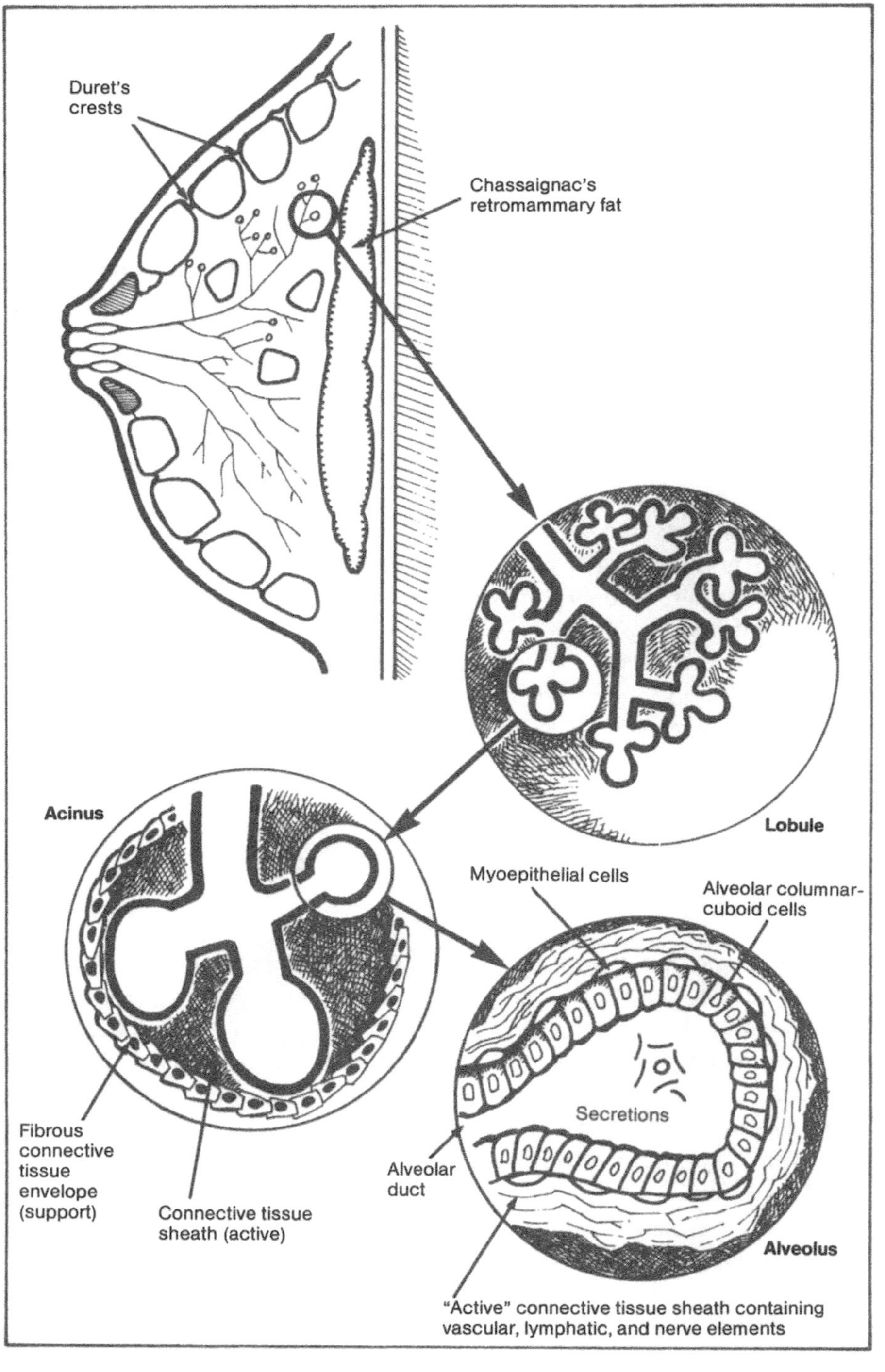

Fig. 114. Anatomic-histologic diagram of the breast

The actual glandular portion, which is epithelial in nature, is composed of branches of lactiferous ducts ending in small rounded alveoli. These alveoli differ depending on hormonal activity. In a resting state they form simple fingerlike endings (alveoli). Under the effect of sex hormones, they become true glandular saccules (acini). Pathologic findings divide the lactiferous segments into three classes:

- Large or primary lactiferous ducts which end at the nipple. Their lumen diameter is greater than the wall thickness.
- Medium or secondary lactiferous ducts with a lumen diameter equal to the wall thickness.
- Small or tertiary lactiferous ducts with a lumen narrower than the wall. They have both intra- and extralobular segments.

The ducts and alveoli or acini are surrounded by a discontinuous layer of flat myoepithelial cells.

The connective tissue of these branchings is not only for support. This mesenchymatous stroma is mainly composed of fibroblasts and plays an active role in glandular development, function, and metabolism, especially in the periacinous sheaths (active connective tissue). It also contains endothelial cells forming small vascular and lymphatic vessels.

Examination Findings for the Lactiferous-Connective Tissue Network

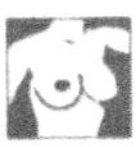

Palpation: Supple. May be firm if turgescent; may form a band or granulation.

Transillumination: Average opacity.

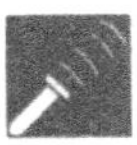

Ultrasonography: Moderately echogenic, average absorbency. Except for pathologic dilation, the ductal lumen cannot be distinguished.

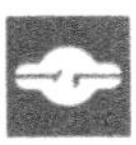

Mammography: Average radiographic density, equivalent to that of water. Contour may or may not be detected depending on the surrounding tissue. Ductal lumen is visualized by means of artificial contrast: galactography.

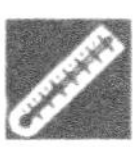

Thermography: Heat production directly related to endocrine activity. Average thermal transfer.

2.1.2 "Passive" Mesenchyma

This is stroma containing few cells, elastic and other fibers, and adipose tissue. It fills out the space between lobes and lobules and separates the gland from the skin and fascia pectoralis (retromammary cellular-adipose layer).

Examination Findings for the Passive Mesenchyma

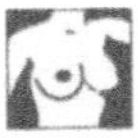

Palpation: Soft tissue.

Transillumination: Highly transparent.

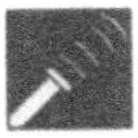

Ultrasonography: Poorly echogenic, poorly absorbant.

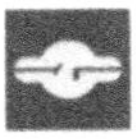

Mammography: Radiolucent unless edematous infiltration which may yield high opacity.

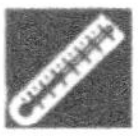

Thermography: Negligible heat production; poor heat transfer.

2.1.3 Blood Vessels, Lymphatic System, Nerves

Since anatomic descriptions vary widely from one patient to another, we will only discuss those essential findings that may be in question during an examination.

2.1.3.1 Arteries

They have different origins. Perforating branches of the internal mammary artery supply the medial part of the breast. The external mammary and subscapular arteries supply the lateral part. The thoracoacromial and highest thoracic arteries are also involved.

2.1.3.2 Veins

The veins form superficial and deep networks. A major part of the normal thermogram is due to the superficial network which may show changes in vascularization and heat production. It is customary to mention an inconstant anastomotic circle around the base of the nipple called Haller's "circulus venosus." Rouviere then says, "this superficial network supplies superficial veins of the surrounding tissue." In practice, the best anatomic map is the opposite side. Even this is only true given a fairly large margin of asymmetry. Deep veins accompany the principal arteries and open into the external mammary veins laterally, the internal mammary veins medially, and the corresponding intercostal veins posteriorly.

2.1.3.3 Lymphatics

The lymphatics have three origins and three terminations:

Origins
- Lobules
- Lactiferous ducts
- Areola-nipple area, the site of a large network draining a major portion of the breast's lymph

Terminations
- Pectoral group of axillary nodes (Sorgius' node is the lowest and most frequently observed)
- Sternal (internal mammary) nodes
- Subclavicular nodes, reached by trans- or retropectoral passage

It is important to note that this distribution is far from strict and there may even be anastomoses with the opposite side.

2.1.3.4 Nerves

Sensory nerves join the superficial cervical plexus, brachial plexus and intercostal nerves. Glandular nerves reach the gland by its posterior aspect and follow the lactiferous ducts to the nipple. They are derived from the fourth, fifth, and sixth intercostal nerves. They intervene in the trophic and secretory functions of the gland, as well as the sensory erectile function of the nipple.

Examination Findings for the Vessels, Nodes and Nerves

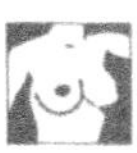

Clinical: During inspection, the superficial venous network is often visible. (Reflected infrared photography greatly increases its visibility. This is the only indication for this technique.) During palpation axillary nodes may be felt without necessarily being pathologic. In this case, they are small, mobile, and painless.

Transillumination: The distinctly opaque superficial venous network is almost always visible. Intramammary nerves and vessels are imbedded in other tissues.

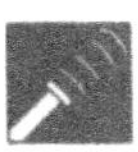

Ultrasonography: Special anatomic and technical conditions or a superhuman effort would be necessary to distinguish the vessels. While they do have structural characteristics similar to those of fluid cavities, their small size makes detection impossible. Lymph nodes, however, if accessible to the transducer have a slightly echogenic lacunar image with regular contours and clearly do not absorb the ultrasound beam.

Mammography: Radiographic density of vessels, nodes, and nerves is approximately that of water. Images of vessels that are visible are due to either atheromatous calcification of the walls or highly or relatively radiolucent surrounding tissue. When the breast is dense, these are usually superficial veins. It may be possible to view deep vessels in a breast lacking in glandular tissue.

Thermography: It is primarily the superficial venous network in the form of variably branched, linear, hyperthermic traces that is viewed. It is normally 2°C higher than the surrounding tissue.

2.1.4 Areolar-Nipple Area

2.1.4.1 Nipple

The nipple is a fibroelastic dermal papilla containing the last centimeter of the lactiferous ducts. It is either projecting or inverted depending on the subject and may be modified by areolar contraction.

2.1.4.2 Areola

This is a zone of variable pigmentation 4 or 5 cm in diameter surrounding the nipple. Large sebaceous glands (glands of Montgomery) produce elevations on its surface. The nipple-areolar reflex causes contraction of its radiating and circular smooth muscle fibers (thelotism).

2.1.4.3 Retroareolar Region

Lactiferous ducts converge here before perforating the nipple. It is particularly rich in connective tissue fibers.

Examination Findings for the Areolar-Nipple Area

Clinical: The nipple is mobile and supple. The retroareolar region is firm and slightly irregular but fairly symmetric around the central axis of the nipple.

Transillumination: The retroareolar region is homogeneous and of average density. Occasionally, it may be highly dense bilaterally in the absence of any disease.

Ultrasonography: The elevated nature of the nipple and areola make for poor transducer contact. They create a false cone of absorption obstructing the underlying areas, particularly the retroareolar region.

Mammography: The nipple, areola, and retroareolar region are highly opaque. Unless the nipple is viewed tangentially, it may form a nodular image with distinct contours making interpretation difficult.

Thermography: Unless inverted the nipple is cold compared with the rest of the breast. Nevertheless, Haller's vascular circle sometimes surrounds it with a tight ring.

2.1.5 Skin

The skin is fine and separated from the mammary gland by subcutaneous fatty tissue but is firmly linked to Duret's crests. It is thicker at the periphery especially along the submammary fold and axillary tail.

Examination Findings for the Skin

Clinical: It is easily mobilized over the fatty tissue during palpation. When pinched, adipose lobules produce small elevations.

Transillumination: The skin's pigmentation slightly attenuates the light beam.

Ultrasonography: The skin is homogeneously echogenic. Its deep aspect is clearly defined by the underlying fatty tissue which contains few echoes and is fragmented by the echogenic crests.

Mammography: The skin has an average radiolucency. A fine, opaque line outlines the breast by a tangent effect. It is less than 1 mm thick (2 mm along the submammary fold and axillary region). At the periphery, sebaceous and sweat glands form small granulations.

Thermography: Normal skin is a good thermal conductor. It can be compared to a black body due to its infrared radiant power characteristics.

2.2 Organic-Functional Variations Related to Normal Sex Hormone Activity

The breast is a target for three types of sex hormones: estrogens, progestins, and prolactin.

2.2.1 Prepuberty

Sex hormone activity is insufficient for breast development. At this stage, the breasts are only represented by a pigmented nipple and areola. Lactiferous ducts are at an infantile stage with no difference between boys and girls.

Examination Findings

Clinical: When palpated, the nipple is supple and underlying tissues have a fatty tissue consistency.

Transillumination: There is no opacity.

Ultrasonography: It is often possible to perform this examination since the nipple and areola are quite supple. Echogenicity is the same as in adjacent areas.

Mammography: A small homogeneous opacity, denser than the surrounding adipose tissue, and less than 1 cm deep can be observed. This corresponds to connective tissue elements.

Thermography: Temperature is low; vascularization is type A.

2.2.2 Puberty

Ovarian estrogen secretion marks the beginning of this period in girls (12–15 years). It is not unusual to see slight, spontaneously regressive, prepubertal mammary development at about 8 or 9 years of age. Adequate progesterone secretion by the corpus luteum occurs regularly (at least three out of five cycles) only 1 or 2 years after menarche. Puberty is characterized by estrogen activity without effective progesterone secretion and, thus, increased hydration of the glandular stroma.

Examination Findings

Clinical: On inspection, the recently developed mammary structures and increased hydration stretch the skin. Skin tone is not yet diminished. Breast consistency is firm, homogeneous or heterogeneous.

Transillumination: Good homogeneous transparency.

Ultrasonography: Tissues are moderately echogenic; the sonolucent interlobular network is strongly marked.

Mammography: Estrogens have increased capillary permeability and resulted in increased stroma hydration. This causes major, diffuse opacity which greatly attenuates the contrasts.

Thermography: Vascularization is generally quite pronounced. The resulting thermal pattern is usually widespread (type B).

2.2.3 Period of Regular Menstrual Cycles (Fig. 115)

Menstrual cycles last an average of 28 days. During the majority of these cycles (at least three out of five) ovulation occurs in the middle and is followed by formation of the ovarian corpus luteum. Progesterone is secreted by the corpus luteum in sufficient quantities and over a long enough period to have an effect on the breast: a complex action both opposing and complementary to the estrogens. Prior estrogen activity is essential for this progesterone effect.

2.2.3.1 First Phase of the Cycle

Several days prior to menstruation, circulating sex hormone levels drop sharply. The breasts return to a resting state: decrease in edematous infiltration of the stroma and regression of the lactiferous network, particularly the acini. This period lasts approximately 8 days and is the best time for breast examination. Such an examination, therefore, should be scheduled between the 4th and 12th day of the cycle (the 1st day of the cycle is the 1st day of menstruation).

Examination Findings

Clinical: The breast is supple and nontender.

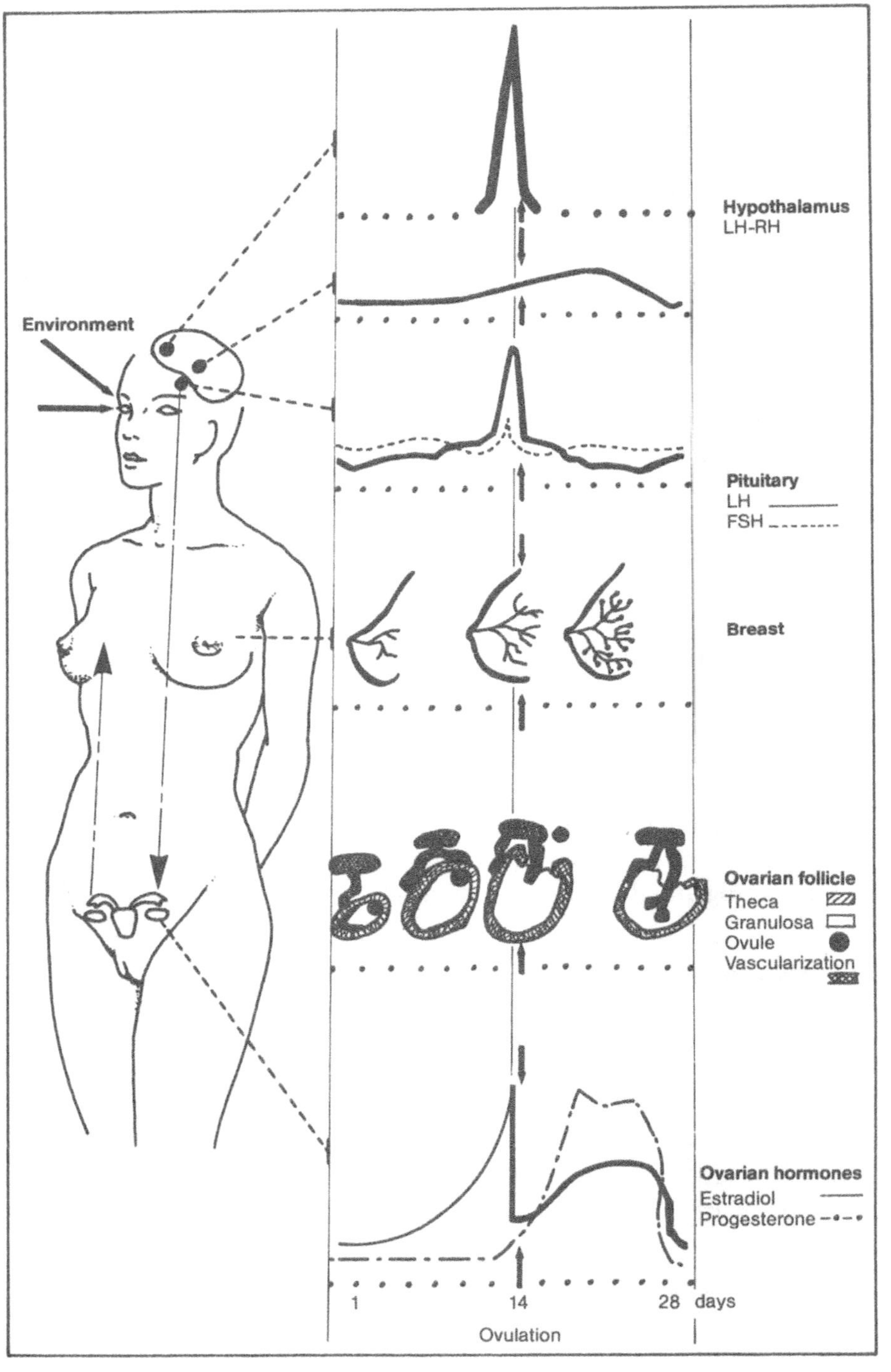

Fig. 115. Hormonal effects on the breast during the menstrual cycle. (From B. de Lignières 1975)

Transillumination: Good transparency.

Ultrasonography: The tissues are echogenic. Nonechogenic interlobular lines are narrow.

Mammography: The tissues are well delinated; contrasts are good.

Thermography: Average vascularization: type A or B.

2.2.3.2 Second Phase of the Cycle

A surge in estradiol secretion between the 12th and 14th days is followed by ovulation. Estrogen secretion continues to increase while the corpus luteum secretes progesterone. The breast, then, is subject to the simultaneous action of both hormones:

- Estrogen activity continues by increasing vascular permeability causing edema and lengthening the ducts.
- Combined estrogen-progesterone activity tends to lessen the edema and reinforce the lactiferous development begun under the effect of estrogen alone. Ductal lengthening is slowed in favor of development of the acini. A slight watery or lactescent discharge at the end of the cycle is not pathologic.

Examination Findings (Compared with the First Phase)

Clinical: The breasts are firmer and tender. Increased pressure at the end of the cycle may force a drop of fluid from the nipple.

Transillumination: Transparency decreases due to cellular proliferation.

Ultrasonography: Tissues are more echogenic due to the acinous growth. Lobulation is more prominent due to the increased sonolucent interlobular spaces.

Mammography: Contours are less defined. Contrasts are attenuated by the increased hydration.

Thermography: Vascularization and heat level are increased by the elevated metabolism (strong type B or D).

2.2.4 Pregnancy and Lactation

2.2.4.1 Pregnancy

Instead of dropping to trigger menstruation, hormone secretion continues to increase and reaches high levels at the end of pregnancy. Changes in the breast that occurred during the second phase of the cycle also persist: glandular development, capillary permeability, and infiltration of the stroma which insure the increase in nutrients necessary for mammary growth.

Glandular epithelial cells undergo change in order to insure their secretory function during lactation. Except for a slight discharge of colostrum that may appear toward the 2nd month there is no excretion before birth. Prolactin levels also increase regularly during pregnancy but their effect on mammary secretion is blocked by high estrogen and progesterone levels.

Examination Findings

Clinical: The breast is increasingly distended. The skin is lined by a rich venous network. Elevations and pigmentation of the nipple and areola are more prominent. Consistency is firmer.

Transillumination: Breast volume and cell multiplication decrease transparency.

Ultrasonography: Echogenic tissues are abundant and prominent lobulation is outlined by connective tissue infiltration.

Mammography: If necessary in early pregnancy, mammography can be performed with special radiation protection. Later in the pregnancy the homogeneous and high density of the breast impede mammographic examination and it is best, if possible, to wait for menstruation to resume.

Thermography: The heat level continues to increase and vascularization usually has a network pattern (type D).

2.2.4.2 Lactation

There is a sharp drop in estrogen and progesterone secretion at birth. Prolactin activity is unmasked and full milk secretion begins in 3 or 4 days. The duration of this secretion is variable. It is maintained by a complex neuroendocrine process in which nipple stimulation by the infant's sucking plays an important role.

Examination Findings

Only palpation and ultrasonography demonstrate any difference compared with the end of pregnancy.

Clinical: The massive firmness of the breast appears dissociated into macronodular elements of average consistency.

Ultrasonography: Milk secretion facilitates ultrasound transmission, which clearly demonstrates lactiferous differentiation into lobes and lobules. Microlacunae corresponding to the distended alveoli are scattered throughout the image.

2.2.5 Premenopause and Menopause

Ovary function decreases and the frequency of inadequate corpus luteum cycles increases to one out of two instead of one or two out of five. This period of premenopause lasts about 10 years. Progesterone activity weakens, leaving the field open to the effect of estrogens, which continue to be secreted.

This endocrine balance is similar to that of puberty except that the connective tissue target has changed. It is not a young dynamic tissue but one marked by opposing endocrine influences over many years. Weary fibroblastic cells give in to the temptation of sclerosis. It is thus a modified heterogeneous tissue subject to the effects of estrogen. Ductal lengthening occurs under altered nutritional conditions. Microcystic ectasia of the acini is often observed.

Examination Findings

Clinical: Mastodynia develops, reoccurs, or increases in intensity and duration. During palpation, consistency is fairly firm and notably heterogeneous.

Transillumination: There may be sufficient sclerosis to create a shadow.

Ultrasonography: Hypoechogenic adipose tissue replaces much of the echogenic lactiferous and connective tissue.

Mammography: Much as the fibrosis does not obstruct it, water infiltration thickens and blurs the tissues. This is incomplete, however, and often only occurs in scattered patches.

Thermography: Vascular type is extremely variable from one woman to another. Residual metabolism is fairly high, giving rise to a strong type B or D vascularization. Adipose tissue, on the other hand, impedes heat transmission. Type A vascularization may be observed if deep veins are more utilized or simply if metabolism decreases.

2.2.6 Postmenopause

In principle, sex hormones are no longer secreted by the ovary. It is the end of menstruation but far from the end of the breast. Fatty tissue, now occupying most of the space, together with the fibrous remnants of lactiferous and connective tissues, is able to maintain breast volume. With increasing age, calcium can impregnate the fibrous tissue and vascular walls.

Examination Findings (Appendix, Fig. 124)

Clinical: Flattening and diminished pigmentation of the nipple and areola are often noted. Palpation reveals decreased consistency.

Transillumination: The adipose tissue is highly transparent.

Ultrasonography: Scattered bands within large hypoechogenic adipose patches.

Mammography: Fibrous remnants are easily studied due to the high radiolucency. Calcifications, mostly vascular, may be observed.

Thermography: Low heat level; type A vascularization.

3 Abnormalities and Breast Disease

3.1 Local Congenital Abnormalities

Only abnormalities of the receptor organ are covered in this section. Abnormalities due to congenital defects in the hypothalamic-hypophyseal-gonadal endocrine system are discussed in the next chapter. An endocrine abnormality in the mother or ill-timed treatment may, however, induce a congenital defect in the local receptor.

3.1.1 Embryologic Review

A band of ectoderm thickens toward the 5th week of embryonic development to form the "milk line" (Fig. 116), which extends from the axilla to the inguinal region. The entire band recedes except for a slight elevation corresponding to the future nipple: the mammary crest which is unique in the normal human embryo. Lactiferous ducts develop during the 6th month of intrauterine life. Animal experimentation has shed some light on the influence of hormones during this embryonic development.

- Androgens injected into the mother inhibit nipple formation (athelia).
- Estrogens stimulate mammary development.
- Progesterone inhibits lactiferous duct formation.
- At the end of pregnancy, insulin stimulates development of the lactiferous duct lumen. This effect is enhanced by prolactin and aldosterone.
- Progesterone stimulates the secretory response.

3.1.2 Anomalies by Deficiency

3.1.2.1 Hypoplasia

Glandular development is interrupted during the last trimester of pregnancy. Hormonal stimulation at puberty and during pregnancy have no effect.

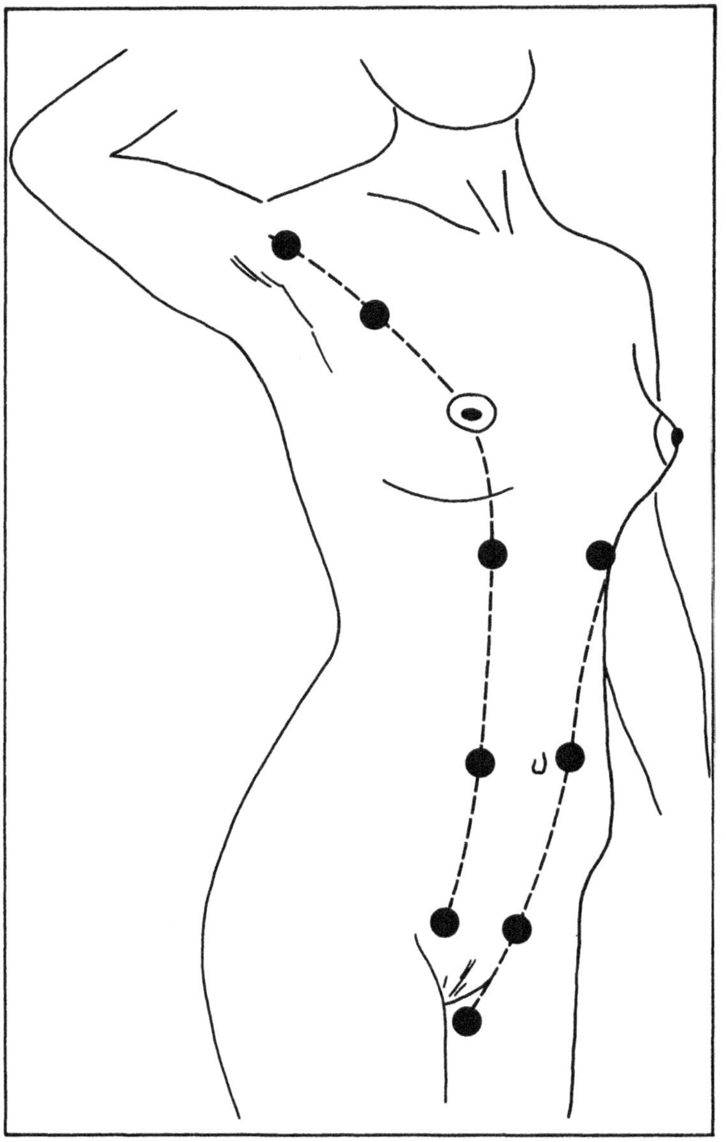

Fig. 116. The "milk line"

3.1.2.2 Aplasia

A disturbance earlier in the pregnancy may result in total absence of the mammary gland. Other malformations are associated: cutaneous and muscle aplasia, bony defects, etc.

3.1.2.3 Amastia

If even earlier, the gland, areola, and nipple (athelia) are all absent.

3.1.3 Anomalies by Excess

3.1.3.1 Polythelia and Polymastia

Involution of the milk line does not occur normally. Supernumerary breasts at different stages of development may form according to the histologic classification of Kéjava:
- Complete breast with nipple, areola, and glandular tissue
- Glandular tissue and nipple without areola
- Glandular tissue with neither areola nor nipple
- Nipple and areola without glandular tissue
- Nipple only
- Areola only
- Simple small tuft of hair

3.1.3.2 Hypertrophy

It is difficult to distinguish between excess hormonal secretion and excessive mammary response to normal hormonal secretion. Certain forms of major hypertrophy with epithelial hyperplasia in the absence of other endocrine abnormalities are indicative of local receptor hypersensitivity.

3.1.4 Asymmetry

Slight mammary asymmetry is normal, particularly during puberty. Otherwise, all types and degrees of asymmetry may occur:
- The volume of both breasts remains within normal limits.
- One breast is obviously hyper- or hypotrophic.
- Asymmetry is due to a unilateral supernumerary breast.

3.1.5 Nipple Inversion

Axial lactiferous-connective tissue elements are too short for the volume of the breast. It may be unilateral or bilateral, permanent or variable with areolar contraction, corrected or not by compressing the breast, and longstanding or detected during changes in breast volume. Nipple inversion may be an esthetic problem and can be corrected by sectioning the axial elements. It is also an obstacle to nursing. When developing unilaterally, it may simulate the retraction of a malignant lesion.

3.2 From the Slight Hormonal Imbalance to the Organic-Functional Anomaly

The mechanism that assures the periodicity of hormonal functioning is powerful. But there are numerous factors capable of interfering and all have certainly not been established: metabolic, constitutional, psychic, gynecologic, climatic, medicinal, etc.

Hormonal secretion may be sufficiently altered to affect the breast with or without a change in menstruation. The breast has its proper receptivity and each cell its own hormonal receptors. This is to say that abnormalities discussed in the previous section are only specific examples and that differences can be observed between women, or in the same woman from one time to another, or on the same day from one glandular area to another ipsilaterally or contralaterally. These variations are the rule, and as long as they remain slight, are not considered pathologic.

By increasing or persisting, however, they may generate anomalies sufficiently significant to be considered pathologic. It is thus a difference in degree of the same phenomenon that determines whether or not it is pathologic and there is no clear line between the two. This is not just a theoretical problem. Strong arguments suggest that these endocrine imbalances play a role in benign and malignant organic breast disease.

3.2.1 Endocrine Anomalies

We will not go into detail concerning the classification of endocrine diseases. Our objective is to try to relate diverse functional anomalies, discovered during breast examination, to a type of hormonal anomaly. It is important to keep in mind that there are many causes of discrepancy concerning hormonal analyses:

- An abnormal quantity of hormone is not always released into the circulation at the time blood is drawn.
- Determination of the functional activity of the breast is still somewhat subjective on the part of the examining physician.
- During breast examination, the actual result of hormonal action reflecting the breast's receptivity is determined; something hormonal analysis does not do.

3.2.1.1 Estrogen Deficiency

Estrogens are necessary both for epithelial and connective tissue development in the breast and for the correct action of progesterone. If the deficiency is primary, breast development will be the same as in the male. When secondary, the breast prematurely takes on the appearance described in the section "postmenopause." Examination findings are the same (Appendix, Fig. 124).

3.2.1.2 Excess Estrogen and Progesterone

When evenly distributed, this hormonal disturbance causes hypertrophy which may reach detrimental proportions (gigantomastia). It is necessary to make the distinction between true hypertrophy and obesity. In the former, the breasts are out of proportion compared with the patient's body build, whereas in the latter the breasts are proportionately large and not considered pathologic.

Examination Findings

In principle, since their structure is not pathologic, these breasts do not present with any particular feature. The increased glandular tissue, however, may interfere with those techniques based on translucency.

Transillumination: The light beam may be completely absorbed.

Mammography: All available techniques should be used in order to expose the film. If the equipment used provides sufficient blackening without excessive voltage increase (less than 30 kV), it is possible to produce a readable image. Use of a grid is especially indicated here.

3.2.1.3 Estrogen-Progesterone Imbalance

If in favor of progesterone, there is little effect on the breast since progesterone requires prior estrogen impregnation. An imbalance in favor of estrogen, however, is frequent and pathogenic. It is frequent, since it may result from estrogen excess either in absolute value or especially by progesterone deficiency. It is pathogenic since it causes an increase in and edema of connective tissue creating painful breast tension.

Causes of this imbalance are diverse:

- All causes of corpus luteum insufficiency: progesterone secretion is too weak or too brief.

- True estrogen excess, spontaneous or therapeutic.
- Menopause and castration. Estrogen deprivation causes hot flashes which diminish with estrogenic hormone therapy. This creates an imbalance unless accompanied by an appropriate dose of progesterone. Menopause and castration do not necessarily cause hot flashes. This may be due to ovarian or exogenous ovarian (adrenal glands, adipose tissue) estrogen secretion. An imbalance affecting the breasts occurs since there is no exogenous ovarian progesterone secretion.

Examination Findings (Appendix, Fig. 125)

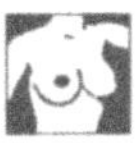

Clinical: Pain is frequent. If the woman is still menstruating this will be in the form of premenstrual mastodynia, which varies in intensity and duration. It may continue into the initial phase of the cycle. Pain is a reliable indicator of estrogen-progesterone imbalance.

Transillumination: Water, which is largely responsible for the mammary tension, does not interfere with the light and thus provides relatively good transparency.

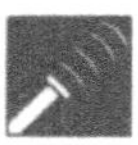

Ultrasonography: The predominant sonolucent intercellular space outlines the structural organization of the echogenic cellular elements.

Mammography: Water is about as opaque to X-rays as soft tissue. The image will be difficult to read no matter what is done especially since contrasts are weak.

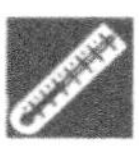

Thermography: The vascularization is highly developed type B with frequent thick branchings corresponding to the elevated heat level of the superficial veins: ball images give the appearance of mimosa. These findings may be intensified during the second phase of the cycle and attenuated during the first phase. They are usually constant, however.

3.2.1.4 Excess Prolactin

This can cause galactorrhea which is a multiductal nipple discharge. It is bilateral and may be clear, greenish, or most often lactescent. It varies in amount from a simple drop appearing at the nipple after compression to abundant, prolonged discharge associated with amenorrhea. Galactorrhea may occur following delivery or abortion. Either one is in and of itself, a cause. Any discharge continuing for more than several months, however, is considered pathologic.

Other than pregnancy, four basic etiologies should be considered:

Medication
Particularly suspect are:
- Psychotropic drugs: reserpines, alpha methyldopa (Aldomet), phenothiazines (Largactil, Noziana)
- Estrogen-progestogen combinations

Trauma or Psychologic Disturbances
It is often difficult to determine the influence of psychotropic medication frequently used in these cases.

Thyroid Insufficiency
TRH stimulates prolactine secretion.

Prolactin Pituitary Adenoma
(Less Frequently Acromegalic Adenoma or Craniopharyngioma)
It is not unreasonable to investigate the possibility of such a lesion even when a medicinal or psychic cause is possible.

The diagnosis is based on two examinations:

1. Radiographic study of the sella turcica:
- Standard profile as well as coronal films
- Coronal and sagittal tomographic sections
- Tomographic sections following pneumoencephalography may be necessary.

These different films are then studied to detect characteristic signs:
- Bulging or ballooning of the floor
- Unilateral floor depression
- Erosion of the walls
- Displacement of the stalk

2. Radioimmunoassay for prolactin:

Normal levels are considered to be from 10 to 25 ng/ml. Normal levels are rare with definite galactorrhea but may be due to poor sensitivity of the assay or the fact that there are two types of prolactin: normal (molecular weight of 20000) and big (mol. wt. of 56000) prolactin. The higher the level, the more probable the adenoma. Prolactin levels may surpass 400 ng/ml.

Examination Findings for Galactorrhea

A diagnosis of galactorrhea is confirmed if the discharge is multiductal and bilateral. The examination will reveal associated signs of estrogen-progesterone imbalance.

3.2.2 Diseases Causing Endocrine Anomalies

The causes of endocrine anomalies which may affect the breast vary in nature and intensity. As we have seen, it may involve a simple temporary disturbance of the hypothalamic-hypophyseal-gonadal axis. All negative influences including psychologic and medicinal may be implicated. Such conditions may persist or generate serious disorders.

The problem may also be actual endocrine disease, in which case any breast involvement is secondary. We do feel it is useful to review the definitions of the principal endocrine syndromes that may be involved. They are listed here in alphabetical order.

Adrenarche, premature: Premature and isolated growth of genital hair.

Amenorrhea: Primary or secondary amenorrhea corresponds to a defect in one of the links of the physiologic chain of menstruation: hypothalamus-pituitary gland-ovary-uterus. A hypophyseal disorder with hyperprolactinemia may lead to an amenorrhea-galactorrhea syndrome. Possible causes include prolactin pituitary adenomas, certain drugs, and the postpill syndrome.

Anorexia nervosa: In the adolescent girl, this is characterized by distorted body image and is accompanied by hypogonadism, amenorrhea, and lowered estrogen, FSH, and LH secretion.

Anovulation: Is a frequent cause of sterility and may or may not be accompanied by amenorrhea. It may be due to a hypothalamic-hypophyseal or ovarian disorder.

Arrhenoblastoma: Ovarian tumor causing amenorrhea and virilism.

Congenital adrenal hyperplasia: Causes amenorrhea, virilismus, and absence of breast development.

Cushing's disease or syndrome: Hyperadrenocorticism. Predominantly affects young women. Head and trunk obesity, asthenia, arterial hypertension, genital insufficiency.

Debré-Fibiger syndrome: Develops in the infant due to mineralocorticoid insufficiency. Death occurs within 6 months without treatment. Treated patients may present with pseudoprecocious puberty.

DeMorsier-Kallmann syndrome: Due to olfactory bulb agenesis and decreased gonadotropin secretion; characterized by anosmia and infantile sexual development.

Endometriosis: Presence of functioning endometrium outside its normal site. Frequent signs related to progesterone insufficiency in the breast.

Follicular insufficiency: Frequent cause of sterility. May result in anovulation. It is characterized by an estrogen deficiency.

Gonadal dysgenesis: Congenital anomaly causing delayed puberty.

Hypercorticism: Due to a tumor or congenital hyperplasia. Causes pseudoprecocious puberty.

Luteal insufficiency: Is frequent and has diverse causes depending on the level of the hypothalamic-hypophyseal-ovarian axis affected. Menstrual cycles are long and irregular; it is accompanied by a significant premenstrual syndrome.

McCune-Albright syndrome: Includes polyostotic fibrous dysplasia, unilateral areas of cutaneous pigmentation (*café au lait* spots) and true precocious puberty.

Morris' syndrome: Testicular feminization or male pseudyhermaphroditism. Amenorrhea, blind vagina, normal secondary sex characteristics.

Ovarian dystrophy: Polycystic ovaries with major luteal insufficiency, increased estrone, and androgen secretion.

Ovarian hyperthecosis: Similar to the polycystic ovary with high testosterone secretion. Causes hirsutism.

Ovarian hypoplasia: Of congenital origin; causes precocious secondary amenorrhea (20–25 years).

Premenstrual syndrome: Painful edema, primarily but not exclusively of the breast. Occurs during the last 10 days of the cycle and is related to progesterone insufficiency.

Primary hypophyseal insufficiency: May cause different clinical pictures. Primary amenorrhea is constant.

Prolactin pituitary adenoma: Represents 30% of hypophyseal tumors. Normal prolactin levels are 5–40 ng/ml (with major fluctuations during the day). With adenoma, levels exceed 100 ng/ml and may even surpass 300 ng/ml. Macroadenomas generate radiologically detected changes in the sella turcica and ophthalmologic signs. Microadenoma diagnosis often requires much more thorough investigation.

Puberty, delayed: Initial signs of puberty are still absent at 15 years of age. Its significance depends on whether the bone age is greater or less than 13 years.

Puberty, precocious: Considered true precocious puberty in the female less than 8 years of age. We distinguish between hypothalamic-hypophyseal true precocious puberty and gonadal-peripheral or pseudoprecocious puberty.

Puberty, pseudoprecocious: Primary and pathologic activation of peripheral glands with absence of pubic and axillary hair.

Rokitansky-Kuster-Hauser syndrome: Congenital absence of the vagina with uterine malformations. Secondary sexual characteristics are normal.

Sheehan's syndrome: Anterior pituitary necrosis following a difficult delivery. Lactation ceases, causes hypoglycemia and progressive multiglandular insufficiency (thyroid, ovary, adrinocortical).

Stein-Leventhal syndrome: Obesity, hirsutism, amenorrhea, sterility. Occurs in young women; considered an ovarian dystrophy.

Telarche, primary: Premature, isolated development of the breasts.

Turner's syndrome: Polymalformation, infantilism, ovarian aplasia.

Virilismus: Causes polycystic dystrophy-type ovarian changes. Bromocryptine may be used to treat certain cases of sterility with virilismus even in the absence of hyperprolactinemia.

Virilizing tumors: Cause secondary amenorrhea with virilism. These include adrenal tumors (adrenogenital syndrome) virilizing ovarian tumors (arrhenoblastoma), and tumors of the ovarian hilus (Leydig cell tumors).

3.3 Mastosis

This chapter deals with benign organic pathology. There is no clear limit between benign disease and functional pathology on one hand and malignant disease on the other. In the latter case, it is probable that some benign lesions represent a precursor state.

The limit between these three types of pathology: functional, benign organic, and malignant organic, remains unclear despite improvements in examination techniques. Difficulties in diagnosis are shared by both examining physician and pathologist.

The most disconcerting problem is in distinguishing between certain benign and malignant diseases. Determining procedure would be easier if this uncertain disease state was more precisely defined and fully accepted by both physicians and their patients. The term precancerous state is upsetting and often needlessly prejudices the future. The term mastosis covers a large portion of benign disease that is not involved. Dysplasia would be a better word if all could agree on its definition.

The examining physician must respect pathologic facts. Unfortunately current examination techniques only function on a macroscopic level. Pathologic and macroscopic features only concur within the general classification of mastosis of which there are many subclassifications. The histologic classification is unquestionably the most significant for the pathologist and the examining physician should be familiar with it.

Pathologic Classification

Mastosis can be histologically characterized as diffuse, bilateral, and polymorphic. These different types of abnormalities may be found separately or combined.

1. Dystrophy involves lesions due to nutritional disturbances of an organ or tissue where a quantitative change in intake is not the cause. Included in this category are micro- and macrocysts, fibroadenomas, and sclerosing adenosis.

2. Dysplasia is a defect in tissue growth resulting in poorly structured tissue. This includes epithelial hyperplasia, fibrosis, adenosis, and mazoplasia (multiplication of the lobules with slight hyperplasia). It is important to note that all transitional stages between epithelial hyperplasia and in situ epithelioma can be observed.

3. Apocrine metaplasia affects ductal epithelium. Cells of the lactiferous duct lining, which are normally cuboid, become large columnar cells with a small nucleus and eosinophilic cytoplasm.

For the examiner and often also for the therapist, correct use of the pathologist's definition of mastosis means:

- Not including inorganic functional states such as increased hydration of the stroma which may develop or recede depending on the hormonal influence
- Not excluding apparently isolated benign lesions such as fibroadenomas or solitary cysts: thorough examination or an additional lesion which later develops often demonstrate other signs of mastosis.

With these reservations in mind, it helps to establish the basic signs of mastosis and a macroscopic classification.

3.3.1 Apparently Isolated Lesions

3.3.1.1 Solid, Well-Delineated Masses

These are generally indistinguishable during noninvasive examination and include: tubular adenomas, lactant adenomas, fibroadenomas (Appendix, Fig. 126), and phylloide tumors (Appendix, Fig. 127).

1. Tubular adenomas are not encapsulated but are well delineated. Their histologic structure is the same as that of normal breast tissue except for excessive epithelial growth.

2. Lactant adenomas develop during pregnancy or lactation. They are also due to excessive epithelial growth but differ from tubular adenomas in that the epithelial tissue forms milk containing alveoli. They may, in fact, represent tubular adenomas modified during pregnancy or lactation.

3. Fibroadenomas develop from connective tissue proliferation. Whether pericanalicular or the more frequent intracanalicular, their growth is slow and may be accompanied by edema. As sclerosis develops, growth ceases and is later followed by calcification.

During pregnancy or lactation, while rare, this growth can be interrupted by infarction which may induce hemorrhagic necrosis. Several authors have suggested the possibility of malignant transformation of fibroadenomas. In the light of the extremely limited number of cases, this possibility can be considered negligible.

4. Giant fibroadenomas only differ from fibroadenomas by their large size and often polylobular form. A high degree of connective tissue edema demonstrated by histologic examination indicates more rapid growth. It is necessary to distinguish between giant fibroadenomas and phylloide tumors.

5. In theory, the phylloide tumor is an intermediate form between fibroadenoma and sarcoma.

Hopefully in the future we will be able to differentiate between those which, despite rapid growth, remain localized and those which may metastasize (primarily to the lung) and must be considered cancerous without reservation.

The phylloide tumor is ten times rarer than the fibroadenoma and derives its name from its histologic appearance: light mesenchymatous proliferation that unfolds like a leaf after sectioning.

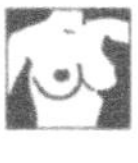

Clinical: Role of age – adenomas and fibroadenomas may be detected in young girls. Since they grow slowly without any functional symptoms they are often detected much later when it is impossible to determine their age. Giant fibroadenomas and phylloide tumors grow rapidly and are detected much earlier. The former are most frequent in young women while the latter (is it merely coincidence) are most frequent during periods of weak or no progesterone secretion: puberty and premenopause.

- *Inspection:* Any superficial mass can cause the skin to bulge. In addition, phylloide tumors may present with signs of their rapid growth: cutaneous edema, increased venous network.
- *Palpation:* The tumor is firm, lobulated, smooth, and mobile. Deep phylloide tumors may appear to adhere strongly to the surrounding glandular tissue. There is no skin fixation. Tubular and lactant adenomas may reach 4 cm,

fibroadenomas 10 cm, and giant fibroadenomas and phylloide tumors 15 cm or more.

Transillumination: The different solid benign tumors are averagely opaque. Their contours are usually easily distinguished from adjacent tissue.

Ultrasonography: Solid benign tumors have a lacunar image with the following characteristics:
- Distinct contours with lateral shadows except for the adenoma whose contour is often blurred.
- Several evenly distributed interior echoes.
- No major change in the beam's intensity. It may be slightly attenuated or reinforced.

Mammography: The opacity is homogeneous with a distinct contour which, in thick areas, is often bordered by a fine line. Its size is equal to that of the palpated mass. Adjacent bands are displaced, never retracted.

Thermography: Only giant fibroadenomas and phylloide tumors, because of their rapid growth, have thermographic features: type C vascularization, localized hyperthermia of 1–2°C.

Needle biopsy: The principle of systematic excision of all palpable masses has certain nuances which can only be justified by the quality of the noninvasive examination. With the false negative being the "original sin" of needle biopsy, it is wise to weigh carefully the indication of this technique and its results concerning the subject of benign tumors.

- *Indications:*
  When excision has been ruled out. This decision to abstain, cytology aside, must have been based on the results of all other techniques combined. Needle biopsy should not be attempted unless the size and site of the lesion guarantee success.
  When excision is being considered. If there is any doubt as to the nature of the lesion, needle biopsy, if positive, will confirm the diagnosis before surgery and may help in formulating the therapeutic strategy.
- When the cytodiagnosis states "benign":
  It is essential that it be significant. A benign tumor will provide abundant cellular material composed of regular and cohesive lactiferous cells. In this case, it may lend support to a decision in favor of abstension.
  Even with good technical reliability, a cytodiagnosis of "benign" should never challenge a previous decision for open biopsy.

3.3.1.2 Poorly Delineated Solid Masses

In addition to sclerosing adenosis, experience obliges us to consider an indescribable entity: the nameless nodule.

Sclerosing Adenosis (Appendix, Fig. 128)

This is characterized by the association of both lobular epithelium and myoepithelial cell proliferation. In a short first phase, this lesion presents as a tumor. Under the effect of myoepithelial cells, sclerosis gradually replaces the cellular elements. Calcifications are witness to the previous epithelial proliferation.
- During the initial tumoral phase, the symptomatology is essentially the same as that of adenomas and fibroadenomas. Age of onset is variable, with a maximum of 30–40 years.
- The appearance changes during the second, sclerosing phase.

Palpation: The mass is firm, irregular, and completely mobile. It may reach 3 cm in diameter.

Transillumination: A small distinct opacity is frequently observed.

Ultrasonography: The pathologic area produces heterogeneous echoes: combination of hypo- and hyperechogenic zones. There is no distinct contour. The intensity of the beam may be unchanged or attenuated.

Mammography: In its tumoral phase, sclerosing adenosis can appear as a solid benign mass: low-density homogeneous opacity, polylobular with fairly distinct contours. It may also present as a zone of somewhat confluent adenosic nodules. In this case, the image will show small, rounded, moderately dense opacities forming a poorly delineated zone. In both cases, disquieting brightly grouped microcalcifications may already be present. During the sclerosis phase, the radiographic image changes and converging fibrous bands appear. Its resemblance to scirrhous carcinoma is striking. Open biopsy is often performed to confirm the diagnosis. The differences are very slight: no cutaneous thickening and no increased central opacity, which is the rule with scirrhous cancer.

Thermography: In principle, thermography offers a hope for differentiation; even superficial slcerosing adenosis should not alter the thermogram. Unfortunately, the quiescent scirrhous tumor does not either and one cannot take a chance on overlooking this possibility.

Needle biopsy: This is only indicated if the evidence is in favor of cancer. If the result is positive, it may help in planning a therapeutic strategy prior to surgery. A negative result, here, is always an indication for open biopsy.

The Nameless Nodule

Occasionally, palpation or transillumination or ultrasonography or mammography will demonstrate a localized abnormality for which none of the techniques is able to indicate its nature or even to confirm it. It is not a problem of classification since we can easily imagine different origins: estrogenic hyperreceptive zone where edema is more likely to develop, localized tendency for adenosis without any distinct formation, scaring as a result of abscess, surgery or trauma, etc. The real problem is in choosing the correct procedure. Prior knowledge of one such etiology may influence the diagnosis and indicate the need for future follow-up.

An isolated warm zone demonstrated by thermography may pose the same problem.

3.3.1.3 **Dystrophic Cysts** (Appendix, Fig. 129)

Not included in this section are the abscess, galactocele, and oil cyst, a particular type of galactocele. A cyst is a closed, encapsulated cavity containing fluid under variable pressure. It is the perfect example of mammary dystrophy. It develops when lactiferous duct obstruction by sclerosis or bending is associated with retained secretions. Even once formed, a cyst may retain the ability to secrete as well as reabsorb. Too much coffee or tea favor fluid secretion (role of xanthines). From the size of the head of a pin to a 50-ml cavity, the cyst is highly polymorphic and frequently encountered. According to pathologists, cystic formations are constantly observed in women after the age of 40 years. Clinically, the maximum frequency is seen after 40 years of age. Oral contraception seems to have lowered this age, however, and cysts are now far from exceptional before the age of 20 years.

There are numerous anatomic forms of cysts:

- According to size and number, contiguity, and communication between several cysts
- According to the mammary tissue: dystrophic or not
- According to the thickness of the wall: up to 1 cm and varying in sclerotic content
- According to the contents: clear, dark, bloody

The development and detection of mammary cysts is variable. Even a large cyst, if not under pressure, is not painful and may go unnoticed during palpation. When a cyst is full, any increased secretion creates excess pressure causing pain and a palpable mass. Use of ultrasound has clearly demonstrated this phenomenon of the clinically "phantom cyst." The role that a progesterone deficiency plays in the development of cysts appears to be well established and the hormonal balance will influence its growth.

Detection of a cyst (or several) should not distract but alert the physician:

- Is there an intracystic vegetation – often benign, sometimes malignant?
- Is there another contiguous or distant lesion – benign or malignant?
- Is it possible to improve the hormonal balance?

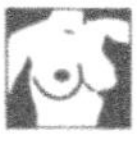

Clinical:

- *Chief complaint:* Pain is often the first symptom. The sharp onset of pain does not correspond to rapid growth of the cyst, but to sudden excess fluid pressure.
- *Inspection:* A superficial cyst displaces the skin and/or nipple.
- *Palpation:* Due to the excess pressure the cyst suddenly becomes palpable. It is firm, rounded, smooth, and freely mobile. The resistance, or transfer of pressure from one finger to another, is inconstant since it depends on the flexibility and thickness of the wall.

Transillumination: A cyst is translucent or opaque depending on whether the liquid is clear or dark. When visible, its contour is distinct.

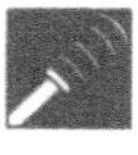

Ultrasonography: This is the best diagnostic tool for cysts. Fluid is sonolucent: no echoes are reflected. Since virtually no ultrasonic waves are absorbed, the beam is relatively reinforced. This produces a particularly sharp image of the posterior wall and increases the number of echoes once through the lesion. A tangent effect at the lateral walls causes integral dispersion of the ultrasonic waves and disappearance of echoes beyond the point of tangency forming a band of shadow. The basic images of the cyst are as follows:

- A Mode: The curve shows a distinct flat-bottomed "U"-shaped interval. The posterior wall is at least as high as the anterior wall. This can be explained by the reinforcement of the beam. Increased pressure on the transducer reduces the size of the interval (flexible lesion).
- B Mode: The lesion corresponds to a lacunar image containing no echoes, with a clearly delineated posterior contour.
- TM Mode: The curve produced by varying pressure on the transducer demonstrates the malleable nature of the cyst.

Mammography: The opacity is homogeneous with distinct contours; rounded or polycyclic in the case of grouped cysts. Since fluid density is equal to that of connective tissue the image is not always discernible. A variable position of the contour may be visualized due to the edge effect depending on the nature of adjacent tissue. Occasionally, the film only demonstrates an increase in opacity without well-defined limits as the contour blends into the surrounding tissue. Only at a later stage can calcifications in the wall be imaged.

Cytography: If, as is desirable, an ultrasound examination precedes mammography and diagnoses a cyst, needle aspiration followed by sterile air insufflation can be carried out. Here, standard mammography is unnecessary. Cystography is more valuable since:

- It shows everything mammography does and it is better for imaging the cyst without its fluid opacity.
- It makes it possible to situate radiologically the punctured cyst particularly in comparison with any adjacent abnormalities.
- It shows if all the fluid has been removed.
- Whatever the radiographic density of the breast tissue it shows the inner cystic wall as well as any intercystic vegitations.

We should add that insufflation has a therapeutic effect by greatly reducing the frequency of recurrence. Why this occurs is unknown. It may be due to the reopening of a lactiferous duct as is often demonstrated by air galactograms.

Cytology: Blackish, clotted fluid containing necrotic cells and isolated nuclei or even sheets of cancerous cells may be aspirated. This is rarely the case and probably represents a zone of cancerous necrosis rather than cancerization of a cyst. At this stage, we can turn to other diagnostic techniques.

Usually, cytologic examination of the fluid after filtration shows "foam cells" and occasionally idrosadenoid and polymorphonuclear cells. Results generally obtained from this type of cytologic study are not taken into consideration for the therapeutic decision and thus do not constitute an argument in favor of its systematic use.

Thermography: Shows primarily a strong type B vascularization since the cyst is often just the local expression of diffuse mastosis. Even without clinical signs of inflammation the cystic zone is often moderately hyperthermic. On the contrary, a large superficial cyst may create a zone of hypothermia, most likely by displacing vascular elements. In general, any thermogram not showing vascularization characteristic of functional hyperactivity is particularly suspect.

3.3.1.4 Lactiferous Ectasia (Appendix, Fig. 130)

This is overall dilation of the ductal tree with pseudocystic dilation of the alveoli generally accompanied by discharge. It occurs during menopause.

Clinical: Unless accompanied by inflammation, the only sign is a slight, thick, somewhat dark-grayish discharge.

Transillumination: A small opacity is frequently observed in the retroareolar area.

Ultrasonography: The lactiferous ducts can be dilated to more than 5 mm. Under favorable conditions, they may appear as tubular or rounded sonolucent images depending on the direction of the section. The pseudocystic terminal tubule dilations may appear as fluid lacunar images. These images can be masked by fatty transformation.

Mammography: Depending on the surrounding tissue, mammograms may demonstrate tubular images of dilated ducts. Unfortunately the appearance is not sufficiently specific for diagnosis. The same is true for the small opaque nodules corresponding to tubular dilations.

Galactography: Injection of contrast medium opacifies the dilated lactiferous network which may have irregular but distinct margins. Opacification of the tubules gives the classic "pigeon nest" image.

3.3.1.5 **Papillary Adenomas** (Appendix, Fig. 131)

This occurs in women during the reproductive years. Only one duct is affected. It is irregularly dilated and contains a 1- to 1.5-cm elongated vegitative formation.

This adenoma develops in the preterminal section of the duct and poses the problem of differential diagnosis with the rare papillary carcinoma.

Clinical: Often the only symptom is a brownish or bloody, elicited or spontaneous monoductal discharge. Sometimes the lesion is palpable: 1- or 2-cm firm nodule situated where lactiferous ducts converge behind the areola.

Transillumination: A clearly delineated opacity, increased by accumulation of dark fluid, is often observed.

Ultrasonography: Signs are the same as for adenomas: fairly regular lacuna containing evenly distributed echoes. This area is difficult to image with ultrasound and only adenomas of at least 1 cm can be detected.

Mammography: Since the surrounding tissue is often dense, the adenoma frequently does not appear on standard mammograms.

Galactography: This technique shows the dilated duct and rounded or elongated lacuna with slightly irregular contours. It provides a diagnosis of intraductal tumor but only histologic examination eliminates the possibility of cancer.

Cytology: Microscopic examination of the fluid is valuable: the sanguineous fluid contains characteristic papillary cellular clusters.

3.3.1.6 Galactocele and "Oil Cyst" (Appendix, Fig. 132)

Galactoceles are caused by retention of milk secretion in cavities formed by lactiferous duct dilation. This milky cyst usually resolves spontaneously or after puncture. It may cause mastitis, frequently resulting in abscess formation. In rare cases it may persist long enough (several months) for oil transformation to occur, which alters some of the examination findings:

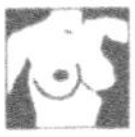

Clinical: Palpation of the galactocele is like that of a cyst. It may be difficult to detect due to retention by the actively secreting surrounding tissue. Oil transformation does not notably alter the consistency of the lesion but palpation may be easier in less distended tissue.

Transillumination: If the surrounding tissue is not too dense, the galactocele is of average opacity with distinct contours. Oil transformation makes it highly transparent.

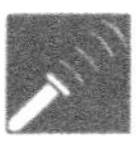

Ultrasonography: The galactocele has all the ultrasonic characteristics of a cyst. Oil transformation of the liquid creates fine, evenly distributed echoes.

Mammography: The galactocele has an image identical to that of a cyst and produces a milky fluid when punctured. Insufflation and cystography are also performed. Since it is lipid in nature the oil cyst is radiolucent. Puncture evacuation is possible but necessitates a low-gauge needle and strong aspiration.

3.3.2 Diffuse Mastosis (Appendix, Fig. 133)

3.3.2.1 General Features

Each of the basic lesions described may occur in large numbers, in different sizes, in one or several patches or throughout both breasts.

Several different types of lesions may also develop at the same time. Such is the very large and indescribable diversity of mastosis and it is amazing that the names Reclus and Schimmelbusch's disease can still be seen in some examination reports. When a large number of cysts or fibroadenomas, or lactiferous dilations are detected, it is easy to envisage a global anomaly of the mammary tissue. Special mention, however, should be made of two particular forms of mastosis: lobular dystrophies and papillary adenomatosis, both of which are dysplasic.

3.3.2.2 Lobular Dystrophy

The lobular portion of the lactiferous duct dilates, forming a microcyst. Epithelial proliferation fills in and deforms its cavities. These cells are capable of secretion. Microcalcifications may develop.

3.3.2.3 Papillary Adenomatosis

This differs from the papillary adenoma by the large number of elements that develop and their small size. The lactiferous segments involved are the fine juxtalobular branches.

Clinical:
- *Functional symtoms:* mastodynia is frequent but inconstant. It makes sense to attribute this to the often associated excess hydration. This seems to be confirmed by the fact that these breast diseases may occur without excess hydration in which case they are asymptomatic.
- *Palpation:* A granular consistency of the breast is highly characteristic. Its overall firmness does not appear to be affected by these types of mastosis. Here again, a total increase in firmness is generally functional in nature.

Transillumination: Total opacity of the breast to the light beam is a good indicator of cellular density or diffuse proliferation. This is a subjective evaluation. Diaphanometry gives a numerical indication of this cellular density, taking breast thickness into account. This method is still in the experimental stage.

Ultrasonography: The lesions are highly echogenic. If the breast is thick, the gain setting should be increased. Microcysts of lobular dystrophy-dysplasia are easily demonstrated.

Mammography: The characteristic radiographic image is fibronodular. It presents as a grill-like structure with many round opaque nodules, 1–4 mm in diameter. This is only readily visible when the connective tissue is fairly dry. With increased functional hydration, the lesions are blurred by the strong diffuse opacity of the water. When present, microcalcifications are relatively large, round, weakly contrasted, evenly dispersed and usually bilateral.

Galactography: When there is a discharge, galactography may opacify dilated acini of the lobules and show small lacunae corresponding to papillary adenomas of the initial lactiferous branches.

Thermography: There is no typical thermographic appearance. It is true that an increased type B vascularization occurs with mastosis. But here, more than in any other case, thermography is particularly valuable since it may be the only technique to demonstrate excessive metabolic activity in one given area. This may represent a vascular change (unilateral type C) or localized hyperthermia.

3.3.3 The Examining Physician When Confronted with Mastosis

Even if able to rule out organic-functional diseases that will respond to treatment, the physican is confronted with a major classification problem. He may be content to record the description and make note of the fact that no sign of cancer was detected. This is, in itself, significant. But, it is important to recognize that at least some breast cancer may be detected early enough if one keeps in mind a sort of hierarchy that goes from dystrophy through simple dysplasia, atypical proliferation, and in situ carcinoma. Despite the diversity of the lesions and their nomenclature this process is well known to the pathologist. When examining a biopsy showing epithelial proliferation he may question the eventual outcome and even hesitate between the diagnosis of proliferation and one of in situ carcinoma since passage from one to the other is imperceptible and both may exist side by side. Is the same approach possible with living tissue? The answer is not obvious; but another question should be asked: are we not obliged to try?

Breast examination techniques attempt to detect the smallest lesion possible. The radiograph of a nodule of several millimeters or small group of microcalcifications or the sonogram showing a tiny absorbant lacuna may lead to an early diagnosis of already invasive cancer. To go a step further, proliferating mastosis, which represents a high local risk, should be correctly identified, treated, and monitored. The great diversity of mastoses can be attributed to two factors: (1) differences between the tissues involved, which each have specific features: enzymes, receptors, tissue structure, etc. and (2) hormonal variations which induce or enlarge the lesions. Such hormonal abnormalities can be corrected or compensated for. Radioimmunoassays make the diagnosis possible but may not concur with the clinical picture for several reasons:

- The assay does not always test for all active hormonal elements.
- Hormone levels normally vary during the day and the month; they may be quite elevated.
- Hormone activity depends not only on its quantity but also on:
  The length of impregnation
  The target's capacity for response
  The synchronization with other hormones

In addition, hormones given for contraception or therapy affect the delicate units that regulate internal hormone synthesis.

This does not mean that hormonal assays are useless, but does show that hormone therapy based on these tests alone is subject to mysterious failures. It would be particularly interesting then to be able to determine the hormonal component associated with a given mastosis. We will attempt to do this without trying to mask the hypothetical nature of such an endeavor.

The more localized the lesion, the less likely a general hormonal imbalance is involved.

Using the headings from the chapter on organic-functional anomalies, we will boldly attempt to establish the relationship between these anomalies and mastosis.

Estrogen Deficiency

When primary, neither glandular tissue nor mastosis develops. If secondary, fibroadipose dystrophy is the only lesion it may cause.

Excess Estrogen and Progesterone

Breast hypertrophy may be histologically harmonious. More often, it comprises highly dense glandular development: this is adenosis. When localized, it forms a tubular adenoma; when diffuse and at an advanced stage, the adenosis is included in the category of diffuse proliferative mastosis: lobular dystrophy and papillary adenomatosis. These are actually forms of dysplasia and imply the possibility of transition to in situ carcinoma. In addition to the possibility of a spontaneous and simultaneous excess of estrogens and progesterone, this condition may result from progesterone therapy for hormonal imbalances. We have seen that it is a progesterone deficiency that most often causes estrogen-progesterone imbalances. Replacement progesterone therapy, here, offers good clinical results. In certain cases, however, the imbalance is due to an actual estrogen excess with or without a clear progesterone deficiency. In this case, it is possible that replacement progesterone therapy will create conditions favorable to proliferative mastosis. This may explain certain failures of progesterone therapy and discourage its long-term use unless the benefits and risks are closely checked.

Estrogen-Progesterone Imbalance

This promotes predominantly connective tissue proliferation including fibroadenomas and phylloide tumors. During premenopause, when breast tissue undergoes sclerous involution, the imbalance favors fibrocystic type dystrophy formation.

Excess Prolactine

During the reproductive years it causes simple galactorrhea with no perceptible anatomic abnormality. During menopause, it results in lactiferous ectasia (or secreting galactophoritis).

3.4 Benign Mesenchymatous Tumors

Some of these are rare lesions but should be mentioned since they may represent a precancerous state or enter into the differential diagnosis of sarcoma. At least for the present, it appears they should be excluded from the category of mastosis.

3.4.1 Common Lipoma (Appendix, Fig. 134)

Solitary or part of diffuse lipomatosis, this tumor occurs more often than is reported inasmuch as its appearance is benign, clear, and distinct. Only a thin connective tissue capsule distinguishes it from simple fatty tissue.

Clinical: This is a soft tumor; its clearly delineated wall is sometimes detected by palpation.

Transillumination: The mass is translucent.

Ultrasonography: It is hypoechogenic with distinct contours. Its contrast depends on the type of surrounding tissue. Beam intensity is unchanged or slightly increased.

Mammography: The lipoma presents as a radiolucent mass with distinct contours, which displaces the surrounding tissue.

Thermography: There is no intrinsic thermal change. There may, however, be either a change in vascularization due to displacement of the veins or hypothermia due to the insulating effect of the fatty tissue.

3.4.2 Fibroadenolipoma (or Hamartoma) (Appendix, Fig. 135)

Fibroadenolipomas are not rare. They differe from common lipomas by the presence of fibrous and adenomatous proliferations pressed against each other within the capsule.

Clinical: This mass is firmer than the lipoma.

Transillumination: It is more opaque or sometimes identical to the surrounding tissues.

Ultrasonography: It presents as a well-delineated glandular zone, different in structure but of similar echogenic density to the adjacent tissue.

Mammography: This technique provides the most characteristic image. It shows the distinct capsule surrounding well-delineated fibroadenomatous patches outlined by the radiolucent adipose tissue ("slice of sausage" appearance).

Growth: Their growth is very slow and excision is optional unless diagnosis is uncertain.

3.4.3 Leiomyomas

Leiomyomas are very rare and may develop from smooth muscle fibers in the areolar region. They may also result from muscular differentiation of the stroma. These are included under the heading of mastosis. They form well-delineated slow-growing tumors.

3.4.4 Abrikossof's Tumor

The physician has little chance of encountering this lesion and even loss chance of diagnosing it. Nevertheless, there is no reason that use of such a beautiful name should be the exclusive right of histologists! According to them, it's a superficial tumor of granular cells forming a thick nodule which often raises the skin. It is benign and ever since its description by Abrikossof in 1926 it has been a subject for debate concerning its nature and origin.

3.5 Carcinoma

The presence of a metastatic and recurring lesion affecting life expectancy is the major preoccupation in breast examination. We will discuss the more or less specific examination findings for carcinoma, first from a diagnostic and then from a prognostic standpoint. Diagnosis of the histologic nature of carcinoma is the job of the pathologist; results of the noninvasive examination may, at best, provide an indication. The histologic classification of Stewart and Foote helps to clarify the macroscopic nature of each type. Lastly, we will consider the problem of early diagnosis.

3.5.1 Characteristic Signs of Malignancy

3.5.1.1 Clinical

History of the Disease

The interview may uncover certain risk factors. Principal risk factors can be classified as follows:

Genetic Factors
Breast cancer of the mother or a sister multiplies the risk by 2 or 3. A family history of other cancers as well as for the patient herself also increases the risk.

Factors Involving Sex Hormones
- Precocious puberty (before the age of 12 years)
- Delayed menopause (after the age of 50 years)
- Late age of first parity pregnancy (after the age of 30 years)

Factors Involving Hormonal Imbalances
- Hyperthyroidism
- Diabetes and prediabetes

Nutritional Factors
- Height (over 1.70 m)
- Obesity (over 75 kg)

Factors Involving Breast Disease
Previous benign disease: Statistics seem to indicate increased risk with fibrocystic mastosis. It is difficult to establish the role of common risk factors in this case. Fibrocystic disease is the best understood form of mastosis and the easiest to diagnose since only needle aspiration and ultrasonography are necessary.

Studies of other types of mastosis are lacking. It has been shown, however, that the risk is greatly increased with intradural adenomatosis and epithelial hyperplasia.

A personal history of breast cancer is a significant risk factor (multiplied by 7).

Age
Ruling out a diagnosis of cancer based on the young age of the patient is unthinkable. Statistical findings may, however, be used as an additional factor in diagnosis. Two types of breast cancer have been described based on race:
- "Japanese" or "oriental" cancer based on genetic factors has a maximum frequency at 45 years.
- "Western" postmenopausal cancer is related to environmental conditions.

Iatrogenic Factors

- The role of reserpine has not been confirmed.
- Excessive irradiation must be taken into account. Statistics showing this effect are based on high radiation doses: tuberculosis patients treated by pneumothorax with numerous fluoroscopy examinations; survivors of nuclear bomb explosions.

Socioeconomic Factors

- Risk increases with socioeconomic level.
- Risk is higher in urban versus rural environments.
- Risk increases with the level of education.

Physical Examination

Even when small in size, carcinoma causes edema and sclerosis of the surrounding tissue thus adding to the symptoms of the tumor itself.

Inspection

The tumor may bulge under the skin. Sclerosis results in the characteristic appearance of *peau d'orange* and nipple retraction. Both are better seen with palpation: when the skin is pinched, signs of retraction appear due to the inextensibility of the peritumoral sclerosis. Inspection should be done with good lighting. The light source should be movable as some small cutaneous depressions can only be seen tangentially.

Palpation

The mass is hard and irregular. It is difficult to differentiate from the surrounding tissue. Adherence to cutaneous and underlying tissues is determined by its mobilization (Tillaux's technique). It is painless on compression. Axillary lymph nodes are ipsilateral. The pectoral group is the first to be affected. Nodes in the supraclavicular group should also be palpated. The nodes are large, hard, and remain mobile for a long time.

3.5.1.2 Transillumination

The mass is highly opaque due to the cellular and blood concentration. Under good conditions, the irregularity of its contour can be distinguished.

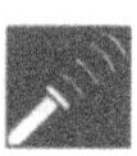

3.5.1.3 Ultrasonography

Cancerous tissue is dense and irregular. It reflects numerous echoes but in all directions. Only a small number are detected by the transducer in such a way that the lesion presents as a lacuna containing a few evenly distributed echoes. The posterior contour is, thus, poorly delineated and is followed by an acoustic shadow: the "chimney"; a hyperechogenic area appears around the lesion. The more echogenic the breast the more distinctly these signs will appear. The lesion may be more difficult to detect when surrounded by adipose tissue.

It is important to look for indirect signs:

- The overlying skin is edematous and less echogenic than in other areas. It may appear thick or thin depending on the setting of the gain.
- The translucent subcutaneous tissue may be decreased by the bulge of the tumor when superficial.
- Echogenic bands corresponding to the surrounding tissue appear forked or split but not displaced.

3.5.1.4 Mammography

X-ray absorption by a cancerous cell cannot be differentiated from that of a normal cell. The suspect nature of the opacity is due to the cellular concentration and edema, which form the radiographic image, and the structural organization of the tissue. The opacity is very dense. The sharpness of its contours, which are irregular and covered with spicules of varying length, depends on the density of the adjacent tissue. A clear halo, due to compressed peritumoral fat, surrounds the lesion.

The tumor may be filled with microcalcifications, which usually have the following distinctive characteristics: small size (10–100 μm), variable shape, strong "brillant" contrast, angular contour, heterogeneous distribution, and clustered at the center, periphery, or even a distance from the tumor.

The mass feels larger than it appears radiologically since palpation cannot differentiate the tumor from the peripheral induration. A large-diameter vessel may be seen adjacent to the lesion. This is usually a vein.

Involved axillary nodes form dense opacities; they are polycyclic and do not have the characteristic central radiolucency of normal nodes. They may contain microcalcifications and produce skin retraction and thickening.

3.5.1.5 Thermography

Increased metabolism related to tumor growth has three consequences:

- Increased vascularization and arterial flow
- Increased localized temperature
- Increased number of calories to be dissipated primarily by the superficial venous network, causing an increase in and hyperthermia of the venous network

Infrared thermographic findings: the thermogram is classified as 3, 4, or 5 based on the following basic signs:

- A localized hot zone of more than 2°C above the corresponding zone on the other breast and 1.5°C compared with the xyphoid reference point
- The association of this hot zone with a morphologically detected lesion
- A hot cuff
- Total hyperthermia greater than 1.5°C of the entire breast
- Total hyperthermia of the entire breast compared with the xyphoid reference
- Asymmetric and irregular (type C) vascular network

Contact thermographic findings:

- Presence of a hyperthermic zone
- Hot nipple
- Vascular anomalies:
  Vascular star with four or more branches
  Vascular circle with a radiating vessel
  Irregular vascularization, "spatula"-ended vessel, aberrant vessel

3.5.1.6 Needle Biopsy

- Patches of malignant cells
- Necrotic debris
- Isolated nuclei

3.5.2 Determining the Prognosis

We list here a number of general elements that can be derived from the noninvasive examination. Identification of the histologic type of carcinoma offers a valuable indication of the lesion's growth potential (see Sect. 3.5.2.4).

3.5.2.1 Based on Radiologic-Clinical Findings

The TNM classification, proposed by the International Union Against Cancer and revised in 1974, is based on the radiologically determined size of the tumor and its clinical features. Five stages are defined (Table 4). Size is determined using the largest diameter, which includes all spicules and any secondary neoplastic zones.

Growth signs are determined according to the Gustave-Roussy Institute of Villejuif:

- PEV 0: no obvious sign of growth
- PEV 1: tumor diameter doubles in less than 6 months. This can only be determined according to the patient's observation or if, for some

Table 4. Clinical classification of breast carcinoma

TNM (classification established by the International Union Against Cancer)

1. T – Primary tumor
   - T0: No evidence of primary tumor
   - Tis: Paget's disease of the nipple with no demonstrable tumor
   - T1: Tumor 2 cm or less in its greatest dimension
   - T2: Tumor more than 2 cm but not more than 5 cm in its greatest dimension
     - T2a: No fixation to underlying pectoral fascia and/or muscle
     - T2b: Fixation to underlying pectoral fascia and/or muscle
   - T3: Tumor more than 5 cm in its greatest dimension
     - T3a: Idem
     - T3b: Idem
       Cutaneous dimpling, nipple retraction, or any cutaneous change other than those mentioned in T4b do not modify the classification
   - T4: Tumor of any size with direct extension to chest wall or skin (other than the pectoral muscle)
     - T4a: Fixation to chest wall
     - T4b: Edema infiltration or cutaneous ulceration (including *peau d'orange)* or skin nodules
     - T4c: Fixation to skin and chest wall

2. N – Nodal inolvement
   - N0: No palpable axiallary nodes
   - N1: Palpable homolateral axillary nodes
     - N1a: not considered to contain nodes
     - N1b: considered to contain growth
   - N2: Homolateral axillary nodes fixed to one another or to axillary tissue
   - N3: Supraclavicular nodes or edema of the arm

3. M – Distant metastasis
   - M0: No evidence of metastasis
   - M1: Distant metastasis present (including distant skin nodules of the affected breast)

Clinical stages corresponding to the TNM classification

Stage 0: Tis
Stage I: T1, N1a
Stage II: T0, T1 or T2 + N1b
Stage III: T3 or T4 + any N,
any T + N2
Stage IV: M1, any T, any N

reason, two mammographic examinations were done at different times without treatment

- PEV 2: presence of inflammatory signs adjacent to the tumor
- PEV 3: massive inflammation: carcinomatous mastitis

3.5.2.2 Based on Thermographic Findings

There is no doubt that contact thermography provides certain elements that aid in evaluating tumor growth rate. It was through infrared thermography, however, that the principles of evaluation, using the basic signs described by the Strasbourg school, were retrospectively developed:

Class Q0: no pathologic sign
Q1: one to three signs except a, b, e, or abg
Q2: three to five signs with a or e and abg
Q3: four or five signs with a and e and abg
Q4: six to eight signs

From Q0, noninvasive tumor, to Q4, inflammatory cancer, the thermographic class corresponds to the growth rate of the disease.

3.5.2.3 Based on Cytologic Findings

The cytologist must decide for himself which classification to use. We will just cite two of the better known:

- Mouriquand's classification:
  Grade 1: Cell bundles
  Rare cytologic anomalies
  Difficult diagnosis of malignancy
  Grade 2: Large cells, isolated and in bundles
  Polymorphic cells with anisonucleosis
  Purple nucleoli (Papanicolaou's stain)
  Grade 3: (most severe prognosis)
  Cells, highly variable in size
  Clear or hyperchromatic nuclei
  Budding, isolated nuclei
- Zadjela and Ghossein's cytoprognosis:
  Based on the diameter of the nuclei (caryometry)
  If more than 80% of the cells have a nucleus larger than 12 μm, it is classified as large-nuclei carcinoma: LN
  In the opposite case, it is classified as small nuclei: SN; this type accounts for 10%–20% of all breast cancer and 90% for those patients still living after 5 years.

3.5.2.4 Based on Histologic Findings

Prognosis may be based on the study of both the surgical specimen and drill biopsy.

Three findings are taken into consideration:

- Histologic type of the tumor (see Sect. 3.5.3)
- Histologic degree of malignancy
- Analysis of hormonal receptors

Based on the evaluation of three parameters:
- Architectural differentiation
- Nuclear morphology
- Number of mitoses

The histologist establishes the grade of malignancy:
- Grade 1: weakly malignant
- Grade 2: moderately malignant
- Grade 3: highly malignant

The different criteria of growth of malignancy including clinical (TNM and PEV), thermographic (class Q), cytologic (grades and cytoprognosis), and histologic (grades) are all remarkably concurrent, a fact that has been verified by statistical studies. Analysis of the receptors provides an indication of the type of response to treatment which enters into the prognosis.

3.5.3 Types of Carcinoma

While a histologic examination is obviously necessary to make a histologic diagnosis (Table 5), the physician should be able to recognize the principle types of lesions and the possibility of certain unusual appearances.

Table 5. Histologic classification of breast cancer (Stewart 1950)

1. Paget's disease of the breast
2. Ductal carcinoma
   a) Noninvasive
      - Papillary carcinoma
      - Comedocarcinoma
   b) Invasive
      - Papillary carcinoma
      - Carcinoma with sclerosis (scirrhous)
      - Tubular carcinoma
      - Medullary carcinoma
      - Colloid carcinoma
3. Lobular carcinoma
   a) Noninvasive
   b) Invasive
4. Rare types of carcinoma
   a) Sweat-gland carcinoma
   b) Intracystic carcinoma
   c) Adenoid cystic carcinoma
   d) Carcinoma with elongated cell, bony, or cartilaginous epidermoid metaplasia
   e) Lipid cell carcinoma
5. Complex types

3.5.3.1 Epithelioma

Noninvasive Epithelioma

A histologic study is almost always necessary to confirm the noninvasive nature (intact basal membrane). It is impossible to predict the behavior of such lesions: definitive stability or passage to an invasive stage.

Suspicion of in situ carcinoma, thus, usually leads to excision biopsy. Even with the lesion removed, a diagnosis of cancer, even if in situ, casts suspicion on the rest of the mammary tissue. The problem may correspond to immunologic or endocrine dysplasia representing a high risk of ipsi- or contralateral cancer.

Noninvasive Ductal Epitheliomas

Supralobular Intraductal Carcinoma, In Situ
This primarily affects small (third order) ducts but may occasionally involve intermediate (second order) lactiferous ducts.

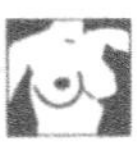

Clinical: The lesion may be completely asymptomatic or be represented by nipple discharge or palpation of a nonspecific nodule. In retrospect, Paget's disease of the nipple appears to have been the first symptom in some cases.

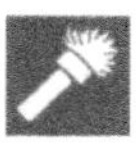

Transillumination: There is no distinct tumoral opacity.

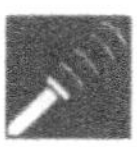

Ultrasonography: A hypoechogenic zone indistinguishable from simple dystrophy may be observed in the case of nodule formation.

Mammography: This technique is not sensitive enough to detect the cellular changes characteristic of in situ cancer. However, calcium impregnates the small areas of necrosis that develop. The resulting microcalcifictions are often the first if not the only sign. They present as irregularly distributed clusters of small highly dense opacities with angular contours.

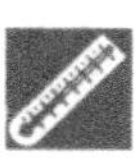

Thermography: No abnormality is detected.

Comedocarcinoma (Appendix, Fig. 136)
This lactiferous duct cancer involves intermediate (second order) units. Its name is derived from the comparison of intraductal secretions to cutaneous comedones (black heads). It remains noninvasive for a long period. Highest incidence occurs between the ages of 50 and 70 years.

Clinical: Symptoms widely vary.
- Pin prick or mosquito bite type pain is often noted.
- Nipple discharge is frequent: serous, purulent, bloody, and sometimes necrotic.
- Paget's disease of the nipple may be the initial symptom.
- It may be a small localized induration (most often situated in the upper half of the breast) which the patient or physician first notices.

Transillumination: The cancerous zone may produce a very slight decrease in transparency detected only by careful examination.

Ultrasonography: At a preinvasive stage, a sonogram will only show slight beam absorption in a fairly limited area with no visible outline. It is only later at the invasive stage that signs of a well-delineated tumor appear.

Mammography: Microcalcifications, which are inconstant, are the only evidence during the preinvasive stage. They produce numerous opacities grouped in clusters. They are highly dense, variable in shape, and density is higher in the center than at the periphery. Often, the microcalcifications have a stone chip appearance. The radiographic image in this case is particularly suggestive of comedocarcinoma. A tumor, usually nodular in nature, develops during the invasive stage.

Galactography: When discharge occurs, this technique demonstrates a characteristic appearance: a lacuna forms where contrast medium is blocked in medium-sized ducts.

Thermography: Unless inflammation occurs, the thermogram is normal during the preinvasive period. Later, it shows evidence of a weakly invasive cancer.

Cytology: Diagnosis can be made by slide analysis of a discharge in the same manner as for papillary carcinoma.

Histology: Pathologic examination of the biopsy specimen confirms the diagnosis. It determines whether the lesion is infiltrating or not. Actually, the difference is quantitative, not qualitative. This type of carcinoma is rarely completely intradural or in situ. The histologist must determine the percentage of infiltration.

Prognosis: On the whole, comedocarcinoma has a good prognosis. Obviously, the weaker the infiltration, the better the statistics. Adenopathy develops only after 50% infiltration.

Papillary Carcinoma (Ductal or Intracystic)

This type of cancer involves first order (large-diameter) ducts or is intracystic. It remains noninvasive over a long period. This slow growth rate makes it possible to combine these two forms. It also makes it possible to distinguish them from papillary carcinoma involving small ducts which have the same growth pattern as ductal carcinomas.

The difference between intraductal and intracystic is more a macroscopic than microscopic distinction. In both cases, the lactiferous duct presents with cystic dilation. In the first case, dilation is moderate and the duct remains permeable. In the latter case, it is more significant and the duct is obstructed. There is a fairly large difference between the two concerning signs and symptoms.

Intraductal papillary epithelioma (Appendix, Fig. 137)

Clinical: Average age of onset is 50 years. It is not painful. Bloody discharge appears. The affected area can be located by the pencil sign (see p. 7).

Transillumination: The affected area produces a fairly well delineated shadow.

Ultrasonography: Resolution is not fine enough to demonstrate the lesion.

Mammography: There is no visible abnormality.

Galactography: Injection of water-soluble contrast medium into the affected duct will demonstrate:
- Moderate dilation of the largest sections of the duct
- Multiple, poorly delineated lacunae
- Occasionally, amputation images

Thermography: The periareolar region is hypervascularized but there is no significant hyperthermia.

Cytology: Slide analysis of the discharge (obtained prior to galactography) often makes the diagnosis of malignancy by demonstrating isolated necrotic nuclei and groups of cancerous cells.

Histology: The surgeon locates the area to be biopsied by injecting methylene blue into the duct using the galactography technique.

The dye should be injected approximately ¼ h prior to surgery. The frozen section usually confirms the diagnosis. The surgeon must then make sure excision is complete. Any breaks detected in the basal membrane are grounds for invasive breast cancer type treatment. The frozen section is often inconclusive and no decision should be made until results from the paraffin sections are obtained.

Intracystic Papillary Epithelioma (Appendix, Fig. 138)
The cyst is a result of ductal dilation due to necrosis and hemorrhage. It contains a bloody fluid.

Clinical: As with a cyst, the lesion develops suddenly. It is a well-delineated, regular, hard, painful nodule. It is striking that this lesion occurs after menopause. Remember the rule: no benign cyst after the age of 55 years.

Transillumination: The palpated tumor is highly opaque since this cyst contains blood.

Ultrasonography: The image is that of a cyst with two particular characteristics:
- It is not completely translucent and necrotic debris may produce several echoes
- Intracystic vegetations may alter the contour

Mammography: Films taken prior to puncture show a well-delineated homogeneous, dense opacity. There is nothing to distinguish it from a simple cyst. It is only when it becomes invasive that spicules can alter the contour.

Cystography: After puncture-insufflation, air contrast usually shows intracystic vegetations.

Cytology: Unlike the case of retentional cysts, cytologic analysis of the fluid from these lesions may yield valuable results.

Histology: Pathologic study of either frozen or paraffin sections confirms the malignancy and determines whether or not the tumor is invasive.

Prognosis: The noninvasive lesion has a good prognosis with limited surgical treatment. The invasive lesion is slow growing: no early recurrence; adenopathy is infrequent.

Lobular Carcinoma, In Situ

This lesion is a subject of discussion by pathologists. It frequently coexists with both dysplasia and invasive carcinoma. It is often bilateral (10% for some authors). The lesion is multifocal more than 50% of the time. Age of onset varies from 33 to 35 years and is thus premenopausic.

Mammography: This is generally the only examination to provide a characteristic image. In almost half of the cases, it shows clusters of microcalcifications of unequal size and angular contour.

Histology: There is no indication for needle biopsy unless the lesion is palpable. (Guided puncture is not impossible but requires complex equipment and is not routinely performed.) It is thus surgical biopsy that provides the diagnosis. Radiography of the surgical specimen may be necessary to confirm the presence of the lesion.

Prognosis: Since there is not complete agreement on the classification, it is difficult to determine the frequency with which this carcinoma becomes invasive. The risk may be between 1% and 4%.

Paget's Disease of the Nipple (Appendix, Fig. 139)

Velpeau, in describing the nipple lesion well before Paget, did not establish its possible link to a deeper breast cancer. Whether English or French, the physician must refer to the description by Sir James Paget. As soon as a nipple lesion is discovered a thorough search must be made for the other component of the disease: underlying carcinoma, in order to detect it in its preinvasive stage.

Clinical: Average age of onset is 55 years. One-third of the cases, however, develop prior to menopause. Pain or pruritis usually leads to discovery of the lesion, which is always unilateral.

- On *inspection,* the nipple presents with a weeping, red, eczematoid lesion. Any nipple eczema resistant to usual treatment should be considered to be Paget's disease. Either cytologic examination of a scraping or nipple biopsy should be done. If the diagnosis is positive, additional screening for the deeper carcinoma is necessary.
  Sometimes the clinical appearance is less evident: several small scabs, slight roughness of the nipple, or a superficial, bright red transverse erosion. Occasionally, the nipple is normal and only biopsy provides the diagnosis. It remains supple and erectile during the principal stage of the disease but may later become retracted.
- *Palpation* may detect the underlying tumor, which is usually nodular and situated in the lower quadrants. Often, it is unpalpable.

Transillumination: This may show a decrease in retroareolar transparency and the opacity of the underlying tumor.

Ultrasonography: Shows signs of nodular cancer forming an irregular lacuna which absorbs the beam.

Mammography: The mammographer should look for three different elements:
- Thickening of the areolar region.
- Elongated, rod-like ductal calcifications primarily in the retroareolar region. They can be observed in all areas. Microcalcifications sometimes suggest comedocarcinoma, which, in certain cases, is the underlying lesion of Paget's disease.
- The underlying tumor which is usually nodular.

Thermography: The disease is characterized by hyperthermia of the areolar region. Additional thermographic signs of the underlying tumor may also be present, but since the lesion is usually slow growing the thermogram is not significant.

Cytology: Cytologic examination of the nipple secretion after scraping may provide the diagnosis by showing signs of common ductal carcinoma and cells characteristic of Paget's disease. These are clear, granular cells with abundant cytoplasm and hyperchromatic irregular nuclei.

Histology: Both nipple and underlying tumor biopsies are studied. Paget cells are found in the nipple. They may be scattered or organized depending on the date of onset, but do not involve the dermis. The underlying carcinoma is either ductal or lobular and often noninvasive. A persistent examination is often necessary to detect in situ carcinoma. The histogenesis of Paget's disease has not yet been absolutely established. It is generally considered to involve ductal migration of an underlying carcinoma to the nipple. Other theories are also supported: the underlying cancer is separate but concomitant to the nipple lesion; it may also involve migration of the nipple lesion.

Prognosis:
- More severe before menopause
- In general Paget's disease rarely causes death
  Long-term survival and treatment depend on:
- Growth of the underlying cancer (palpable or not)
- Presence or absence of adenopathy

Invasive Epitheliomas

"Noninvasive" Carcinoma Discovered by Histologic Examination

Histologic examination of each of the "noninvasive" carcinomas described above may detect signs of involvement. Determining the degree of involvement may give an idea of the seriousness of the disease but within such a large margin that it is hardly worth considering.

Clinical Forms of Clinically Invasive Carcinoma

These clinical forms, even more so than the histologic types of cancer, depend on the stroma reaction, which is at least partially dependent on the body's immunologic competence. Described below are four types of stroma reaction in decreasing order and thus of increasing gravity followed by a discussion of advanced cancer.

Scirrhous Carcinoma (Appendix, Fig. 140)
These are characterized by the greatest degree of stroma reaction. Modern examination techniques, mammography in particular, have remarkably enlarged the classic clinical picture in which sclerosis invades the skin, nipple, and deeper tissues, causing fixation to the thoracic wall and retraction with progressive disappearance of the cancerous glandular tissue. The scirrhus is always cancerous and causes a strong sclerotic reaction. It may be small, however, and the sclerosis may have no specific clinical expression.

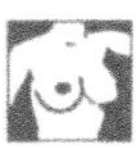

Clinical: The fibrous reaction causes cutaneous retraction (dimpling, then *peau d'orange*) nipple retraction, and early fixation to the skin and chest wall. The cancer, its spicules, and the stroma reaction are all indistinctly included in the palpated mass. It is hard, has an irregular surface, and rapidly loses its mobility.

Transillumination: The lesion is somewhat diffusely opaque.

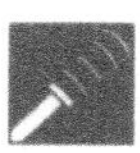

Ultrasonography: The tumoral lacuna is poorly defined but the beam is clearly absorbed. The dermis is distinctly thickened.

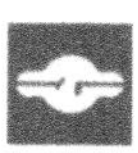

Mammography: The tumoral opacity is radiographically smaller than the palpated mass. It is highly dense and poorly delineated. Spicules of varying length radiate from the surface. It is impossible to determine whether this is purely sclerosis or if neoplastic cells infiltrate between the spicules.

Cancerous-type microcalcifications fill the center and/or periphery of the tumor. Adipose tissue surrounding the lesion forms a clear halo. Diagnosis of a solitary stellate image may be difficult. While it is easy to eliminate superimposition by using at least two views, differential diagnosis of a benign sclerous process, particularly sclerosing adenosis, is difficult. Unlike carcinoma, the latter does not show increased central opacity. It does, however, often present with suspicious microcalcifications.

Thermography: The thermogram is that of a slow-growing carcinoma.

Needle biopsy: This can make the diagnosis. Since precise localization for the aspiration is difficult, there is a certain risk of false-negative results. It can only be justified if non-surgical therapy is proposed. When surgery is considered, a minimum of tumor excision with histologic examination is the rule regardless of the results from the needle biopsy. When results of the needle biopsy are confirmed it can be said that it was unnecessary. On the contrary, a false-negative runs the risk of delayed therapy.

Histology: A predominance of sclerosis may make interpretation difficult, particularly for frozen sections. Under these conditions, it is often impossible to make a definite diagnosis particularly concerning sclerosing adenosis. This is when the pathologist must show his "cool," despite the understandable impatience of the surgeon, and delay his answer until after the paraffin sections have been studied.

Prognosis: As a rule, it shows moderate growth based on the general principles of breast cancer.

Nodular Carcinoma (Appendix, Fig. 141)
Nodular carcinomas only differ from scirrhous tumors in that their stroma reaction is less intense. Our examination techniques have a hard time differentiating between the cancerous and healthy tissue.

Clinical: Clinical signs are generally the same as those of scirrhous carcinoma. For similar growth rates, however, signs of retraction occur later here. The retroareolar localization is a special case: nipple retraction is the initial sign since the tumor is difficult to palpate.

Transillumination: The lesion is opaque.

Ultrasonography: Typical signs of malignancy are demonstrated (irregular lacuna, beam absorption, cutaneous thickening).

Mammography: The tumoral opacity is highly dense, homogeneous, and polycyclic. Its contour appears distinct but close examination will show it to be blurred and covered by fine spicules. Some spicules are long and reach the nipple and skin, causing both to retract and the skin to thicken. As with the scirrhus, it is surrounded by a clear fatty halo. Calcifications can develop. They are large, of low density, and have a striped appearance. Typical cancerous microcalcifications may also appear.

Thermography: Vascular changes and thermal level indicate moderate growth rate.

Needle biopsy: Three-dimensional localization of the lesion is relatively easy and the results are more reliable than for the scirrhus.

Diffuse Carcinoma (Appendix, Fig. 142)
All barriers are broken and neoplastic elements course throughout the breast in an irregular manner.

Clinical: The affected part of the breast presents as a diffuse thickening with cutaneous *peau d'orange* appearance. Axillary adenopathy is usually present.

Transillumination: The entire breast is highly opaque.

Ultrasonography: The glandular tissue is thick and dissociated by edema. Patches of scattered absorption may be observed in any area.

Mammography: The breast is highly opaque, infiltrated with barely perceptible contrasts. The bands are thickened, covered with spicules, and concentric to the curvature of the overlying skin.

Thermography: Hyperthermia and hypervascularization indicate a rapidly growing lesion.

Needle biopsy: While localization of a lesion is impossible, the diffuse nature is such that results are usually positive.

Prognosis: Poor.

Inflammatory Carcinoma (Appendix, Fig. 143)

Not long ago, one referred to carcinomatous mastitis of pregnancy or lactation. Today, all statistics considered, this is inflammatory carcinoma with a maximum incidence during the 5th decade. It is characterized by neoplastic invasion of the dermal lymphatics. All histologic types of cancer may be represented.

Three factors define inflammatory carcinoma: the clinical appearance of inflammation, cutaneous lymphatic invasion, and the extremely poor prognosis. While the last two points are firmly linked, the same is not true for the first: the inflammatory appearance is the most striking and obvious but not the most significant. Retrospective studies have shown that inflammatory type cancer without cutaneous lymphatic involvement may have a 5-year survival rate (14% for the Mayo Clinic). They also show that cutaneous lymphatic involvement with no clinical sign of inflammation (clinically occult inflammatory carcinoma) has as poor a prognosis as when clinical signs of inflammation are present.

Breast examination may in certain cases distinguish between:

- The classic type with inflammatory signs extending beyond the tumor to more than one-third of the cutaneous surface of the breast
- Clinically similar types that may not have the cutaneous lymphatic involvement:
  Localized inflammation of the skin overlying a superficial carcinoma
  Cutaneous inflammation secondary to a cancerous skin ulceration

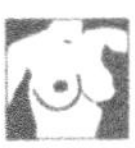

Clinical: The skin is erythematous and slightly edematous (*peau d'orange*), the nipple is retracted, and the breast is painful. The tumoral mass is usually detected by palpation. There is a high incidence of axillary metastases.

Transillumination: The tumor, but not necessarily the entire gland, is opaque.

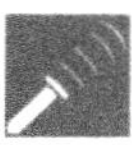

Ultrasonography: Skin thickening and edematous dissociation of the tissues can be added to the characteristic signs of malignancy.

Mammography: Compression is difficult because the breast is edematous and painful. Overall breast opacity is greatly increased. The tumoral opacity and even malignant microcalcifications can still usually be detected.

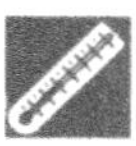

Thermography: This shows major, class 5 hyperthermia of the entire breast.

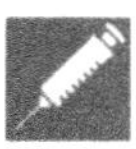

Needle biopsy: One may hesitate to use a needle in this case and the risk of false-negatives is not negligible.

Histology: Since surgery is prohibited due to the risk of explosive metastatic spead, three other approaches are suggested:

- Drill biopsy for which the local consequences are less serious
- Cutaneous biopsy under local anesthesia, which will show the dermal lymphatic involvement
- Axillary node biopsy is possible in the absence of axillary inflammation and provides a reliable diagnosis

Common inflammatory mastitis is the main differential diagnosis. It is rare unless lactation or another cause is evident. The sedimentation rate rises with inflammatory carcinoma but leukocytosis is little changed. A therapeutic test using antibiotics may be determinant but must be rigorously judged since it is not unusual to see the signs of inflammatory carcinoma regress for several days.

Prognosis: Extremely poor: average survival does not exceed 8 months. The prognosis is less favorable before the age of 35 years.

Advanced Carcinoma

Breast carcinomas with poor prognoses usually develop more slowly. Both the tumor and sclerosis develop together. The mass fixes to the skin, nipple, and chest wall. Lymphatic diffusion progresses from low to high axillary groups followed by supraclavicular nodes. Neoplastic dissemination also involves the dermal lymphatics, where it forms small permeation nodules. This occurs without the severity of inflammatory carcinoma. The growing tumor may cause skin ulceration. Skin involvement with hard reddish patches is characteristic of Velpeau's "breast-plate" carcinoma. Lastly, the scirrhus may prolong the sclerosing process that seems to block malignant growth which is remarkably slow. Metastases may appear from the beginning of the disease. Their dissemination and growth obviously increase during the time the disease goes unchecked. Most frequent sites are: the lungs, pleura, bone, liver, brain, ovaries, and choroid.

Special Histologic-Clinical Forms

Invasive Lobular Carcinoma (Appendix, Fig. 144)

This is the extension of in situ lobular carcinoma and is clearly distinguished by the pathologist.

Clinical: The lesion is generally poorly delineated, forming an irregular mass which may cause retraction. Lymph node metastases occur at a much later stage.

Transillumination, ultrasonography, and mammography demonstrate nonspecific signs of carcinoma. Mammography does show microcalcifications of the in situ lesion which indicate the risk or presence of multifocal (50% of cases) and bilateral (10%–20%, synchronous or asynchronous) lesions.

Prognosis: It is relatively good since the 5-year survival rate, with and without adenopathy, is 75%.

Tubular Carcinoma

Tubular carcinoma is termed "well-differentiated carcinoma" by the WHO, and is characterized by pseudoductal, epithelial proliferation and a high degree of stroma reaction. It develops after the age of 25 years and up to the age of 79 years. There is no particular sign or symptom to distinguish it from other ductal carcinomas with sclerosis prior to histologic study. It is not, however, a simple histologic curiosity since it is characterized by a relatively good prognosis: late-stage lymph node and other metastases. It may also be particularly difficult to distinguish from sclerosing adenosis.

Medullary Carcinoma (Appendix, Fig. 145)

This type of cancer strikes young as well as older women. It is well delineated and histologic examination reveals patches of necrosis and numerous lymphocytes. It is bilateral in 10% of the cases.

Clinical: The palpated tumor is regular, rounded, and usually large (5 cm). Since it is not indurated and thus not detected until a later stage, attachment to the skin and adenopathy are frequently detected.

Transillumination: The lesion is opaque.

Ultrasonography: Well-delineated lacuna containing evenly distributed echoes. Beam intensity is only slightly altered. Sonographic appearance is similar to that of adenofibroma.

Mammography: The tumoral opacity is dense, homogeneous, and well delineated with a distinct, dented contour. Stroma reaction at one point along the lesion's periphery forms a radiopaque band with a "comet-tail" appearance. Either skin thickening or nipple retraction will be observed, depending on the direction of this connective tissue fibrosis.

Thermography: Shows signs of a lesion with moderate growth.

Needle biopsy: Provides a more reliable diagnosis in that localization of the lesion by palpation is usually easy.

Prognosis: Despite a moderate growth rate, its clinical features make for a late diagnosis so that its prognosis does not differ from that of overall breast cancer.

Colloid Carcinoma (Appendix, Fig. 146)
Abundant mucus-secreting cells characterize the lesion. Histologic identification is sometimes difficult since all types of well-differentiated carcinoma can secrete mucin. Colloid carcinoma does, however, have distinct features on examination.

Clinical: The lesion develops after menopause. It is firm, resistant, well delineated, and mobile when palpated. Lymph node metastases are late to develop.

Transillumination: The tumor is not visible.

Ultrasonography: Only slightly absorbant and well delineated, the lesion does not appear suspect.

Mammography: The mammogram is also falsely reassuring. It shows a round, homogeneous opacity bordered by a "safe" clear line. Calcifications may fill the tumor.

Needle biopsy: The benign nature of a tumor must always be proven at any age, particularly after menopause. Colloid carcinoma is the perfect example.

Prognosis: Results are relatively good with treatment. When radiotherapy alone is used the radiographic image may persist even after effective treatment.

Rare Histologic Types

Even the best-advised physician has little chance of becoming involved in the complexities of histogenesis. It is best to wait for the firm conclusion of the specialists, who remain undecided. Nevertheless, even if rare, the physician should be aware of these basic types that are difficult for the pathologist to classify.

Carcinoma with Metaplasia
Sweat gland, apocrine- or idrosadenoid-type carcinoma is so called for its histologic resemblance to axillary sweat glands: large cells with acidophilic cytoplasm and small nuclei. Classification and isolation of this lesion is a question for debate since apocrine metaplasia is frequently observed in the breast aside from all neoplasia. Prognosis is better than for overall breast cancer.

Epidermoid carcinoma: Epidermoid metaplasia sometimes accompanies certain types of carcinoma but has, in rare cases, been detected as a separate entity.

These have been postmenopausal cancers with no special clinical or prognostic features.

Carcinoma with osteocartilagenous metaplasis is extremely rare and is considered by some to be a form of sarcoma.

Prognosis is very poor: early and frequent metastases.

Lipid Carcinomas (Lipid Secreting, Histiocytoid)
Histologic examination shows cells with cytoplasm high in fat content. Average age of onset is in the 6th decade. The mass is poorly delineated and with no induration. Local (lymph node) and distant metastases are frequent.

Prognosis: Very poor: no survival after 2 years.

Adenoid Cystic Carcinoma
This rare neoplastic lesion occurs in pre- or postmenopause. It is fairly well delineated and contains cysts of different sizes filled with an amorphous substance. Diagnosis is impossible without histologic examination. The mass is often painful. Ultrasonography may show a centrally located cyst.

Prognosis: Relatively good. Only few metastases have been reported but local recurrence is possible.

3.5.3.2 Sarcoma

Solid Tumor (Appendix, Fig. 147)

Solid tumors are 100 times less frequent than epitheliomas. This mesenchymatous carcinoma is histologically quite variable due to the high degree of transformation of the affected tissue, particularly active connective tissue rich in histiocytes. Except the case where bony tissue is present and detected by mammography, it is the pathologist who determines the predominant tissue in this heterogeneous tumor: liposarcoma, leiomyosarcoma, fibrosarcoma, and undifferentiated sarcoma. Onset occurs between the ages of 13 and 84 years.

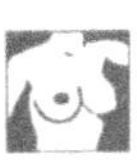

Clinical: The tumor is usually painless. Adjacent tissue changes, especially skin and nipple retraction, occur at a late stage. Thus, it is relatively large when detected and may even raise the skin. It is firm, well delineated, and even fairly smooth. The overlying skin is rarely red. Axillary adenopathy is rarely detected.

Transillumination: Opacity of the tumor varies depending on its size and the surrounding tissue.

Ultrasonography: Lacuna with distinct regular contours; heterogeneous with possible small sonolucent areas corresponding to cystic collections. The beam is clearly attenuated.

Mammography: The opacity is dense and hmogeneous. Its contour is relatively even but may be blurred in spots. Special elements, particularly bony, may be identified.

Thermography: The thermogram is not distinctive and is analyzed in the same manner as are all other neoplastic diseases.

Prognosis: Maximum survival does not exceed 5 years.

Hemangioendothelioma (Appendix, Fig. 148)

This rare vascular tumor has variable malignant potential. It may appear clinically and histologically benign or be highly invasive.

Clinical: It occurs primarily in young women. It presents as an irregular poorly delineated, supple, and mobile tumor. Overlying skin may be altered especially if the lesion is superficial: bluish coloration or ecchymosis. Lymph node metastases are rare.

Trasillumination: The mass is distinctly opaque.

Ultrasonography: Angiomatous cavities are sonolucent. The lesion may also have a high degree of solid proliferation with sonographic signs characteristic of carcinoma.

Mammography: There is no characteristic image. Large calcifications may be detected.

Histology: Examination may show signs of a benign capillary angioma. Even if no suspect areas are detected, the possibility of malignant transformation is always to be considered.

Prognosis: Is variable and may be very poor. The average survival rate is approximately 3 years.

Lymphoma

This infiltration of lactiferous ducts and lobules by lymphomatous cells is diffuse and in one-fourth of the cases, bilateral.

Diagnosis can only be made by histologic examination, which, depending on cell size, distinguishes:

- Well-differentiated, lymphocytic lymphosarcoma
- Poorly differentiated, lymphoblastic lymphosarcoma (or reticulosarcoma)
- Large polymorphic cell, histiocytic sarcoma

A thorough systematic examination is necessary to confirm the primary nature of the breast lesion.

3.5.3.3 Secondary Malignant Breast Lesions

These are extremely rare, comprising only slightly more than 1% of all breast carcinoma. The longest series, published by Hadju and Urban, is based on 51 cases. The main primary lesions in decreasing order of frequency are:

- Malignant lymphoma (lymphosarcoma, reticulosarcoma, Hodgkin's disease)
- Malignant melanoma
- Lung carcinoma
- Myosarcoma
- Ovarian carcinoma

In one-third of the cases, the primary lesion is not detected. One breast may be the site of metastases from carcinoma of the other breast.

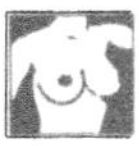

Clinical, ultrasonography, mammography: The lesion is well delineated, nodular, or multinodular.

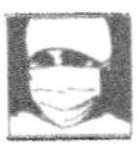

Histology: The secondary nature of the lesion can only be determined on paraffin sections.

3.5.3.4 Occult Carcinoma (False Negatives)

Carcinoma that goes undetected by all examination techniques underlines the limits of breast examination. At times we all make a retrospective diagnosis of cancer after an examination has yielded false-negative results. More often the lesion goes undetected by one particular technique due to a specific weak spot; hence the justification for use of several techniques during any one examination. Even when this is possible, the performance of each should be improved. Before this can be accomplished, it is necessary to analyze the causes of such failure.

Carcinoma Undetected by the Clinical Examination

Inspection: There is no cutaneous-nipple change: no retraction, dimpling, pathologic coloration: noninvasive carcinoma.

Palpation: There is no lump: diffuse cancer; the lump is too small, too deep, or too soft compared with the size and consistency of the breast: in situ or early-stage carcinoma, intraductal or retroareolar carcinoma, comedo-carcinoma, etc.

The tumor is masked by a benign lesion: fibroadenoma, cyst.

Carcinoma Undetected by Transillumination

- The lesion is too small compared with the breast thickness. The light diffuses to the point where no discernible tumoral contrast is produced, even during a thorough examination with changes in the incident beam intensity.
- The breast itself is highly mastosic with an overall opacity to light approaching that of carcinoma.
- The lesion is diffuse. Even if opaque, it is difficult to distinguish during this subjective examination. Diaphanometry will undoubtedly improve the examination in this case.
- The lesion is not in itself opaque: colloid, papillary, and comedocarcinoma.

Carcinoma Undetected by Ultrasonography

- The lesion is too small for the resolution capacity of the unit. While under exceptional conditions breast cancer the size of 1 mm has been detected, suggestive images are rarely obtained if the lesion is under 6 mm.
- The lesion is inaccessible to ultrasonography. It is too deep or retroareolar.
- The lesion is accessible but was not scanned. This occurs fairly often with manual transducers. The latter is primarily used for palpable lesions while automatic transducers examine the entire breast volume.
- The sonographic image of the lesion is not suspect. This is the case of noninvasive and diffuse lesions, tubular carcinoma, lymphoma, etc.
- The lesion is in a weakly echogenic zone. It is a question of contrast: The same lesion can go undetected in a fatty breast and create a distinct image in a highly echogenic breast.
- The lesion is masked by a benign tumor.

Carcinoma Undetected by Mammography

- The lesion is not imaged. This can generally be avoided by a thorough technique. Some areas are more difficult to image: submammary fold, periphery of the gland, in a thin woman, and inner portion of the medial quadrants.
- The lesion does not contrast radiographically with the adjacent tissue: It is too small or not dense enough (diffuse and papillary carcinoma) or the surrounding tissue is highly dense (mastosis and excess hydration).

- The lesion is masked by an adjacent benign tumor.
- The lesion is visible but presents as a benign lesion: nodular or colloid carcinoma simulating a cyst or fibroadenoma; sarcoma simulating a phylloide tumor; scirrhus simulating a common fibrous process.

Carcinoma Undetected by Thermography

Use of thermography alone for diagnostic purposes is extremely disappointing to say the least. That breast carcinoma may not cause thermographic change is not to discourage use of the technique. (Better for the patient that the tumor be cold.) The role of thermography should be to follow the growth or regression of a lesion. This technique can also be credited, in certain cases, with detection of a change in local metabolism where no other method has demonstrated a morphologic abnormality.

We will limit the thermographic false-negatives to those cases where, for anatomic reasons, the technique fails to demonstrate a local thermal change:

- The lesion is very deep or separated from the overlying skin by fatty tissue, which is a poor conductor.
- Thermal emission of the skin is altered by edema or dermatosis.

Carcinoma Undetected by Needle Biopsy

Three causes are possible:

- The needle falls outside the tumor. This method should be abandoned unless the lesion can be precisely localized.
- The needle falls within the tumor but the aspirate contains too few cells (blood, sclerosis).
- The aspirate is of good quality but cytologic examination is insufficient for diagnosis.

Carcinoma Undetected by Histologic Examination

Here again are three causes:

- Cancerous tissue is not included in the surgical specimen. This error should be avoided by carefully controlled biopsy technique and especially by regular use of specimen radiography for nonpalpated lesions.
- The lesion is within the specimen but not on the slide. The diagnosis is sometimes only made when the pathologist insists on additional sections.
- The lesion is on the slide but is not diagnosed. This is more likely to occur with frozen sections of certain lesions. It is best, then, not to place the weight of the examination entirely on this one procedure.

3.5.3.5 False Appearances of Carcinoma (False Positives)

False-positive results of a method are often the source of unnecessary expenses required by additional examination. The consequences may be disastrous if the technique is determinant as is the case with frozen-section diagnosis.

Clinical False Positives

- A benign tumor can be hard and irregular (fibroadenoma)
- Papillary adenoma may cause bloody discharge
- A benign nipple lesion may mimic Paget's disease
- Infection may simulate inflammatory carcinoma

Transillumination False Positives

The problem does not arise since a diagnosis of carcinoma can never be based on this examination alone. Some benign lesions do present as distinctly opaque: dark fluid-filled cysts; fibroadenoma in a small breast with excess hydration.

Mammographic False Positives

- The contour of a benign tumor opacity is difficult to distinguish due to superimposition of adjacent tissue.
- Superimposition of different bands, especially if sclerotic, may create a converging stellate image. Analysis of two views usually avoids this error.
- Sclerosing adenosis with its converging bands and microcalcifications can mimic carcinoma. Distinctive signs, particularly the lack of central opacity, rarely lead to a firm diagnosis of benign nature.
- Benign and malignant microcalcifications generally have distinctive features. Benign processes may have intermediate appearances, making it impossible to eliminate a diagnosis of carcinoma.
- Cutaneous thickening due to edema may be caused by local inflammation.

Thermographic False Positives

Thermography only deceives those who overestimate its capabilities. While it is true that carcinoma may cause hypervascularization or hyperthermia, one does not necessarily equal the other. There are many other causes: distrophic, functional, and inflammatory processes. There are, however, authentic thermographic false positives: isolated thermographic anomalies which are ultimately shown to be nonpathologic.

Histologic False Positives

We have already considered the problem of misleading appearances such as in frozen sections of sclerosing adenosis. One of the major problems is when the pathologist is forced to give a "yes" or "no" answer. Better examination techniques detecting more questionable lesions have only increased the number of these situations. Progress will be made when these intermediate states are accepted by diagnosticians as they are by therapists.

3.5.3.6 Treated Carcinoma

Direct Consequences of Curative Treatment

Surgery

Two different circumstances require examination after surgery:

In the days or weeks following surgery, examination will confirm that the entire lesion was removed. Radiography of the anatomical specimen during surgery may indicate a need for additional confirmation particularly in the case of multifocal lesions. Examination is difficult due to the pain, hematoma, and skin thickening. It should be limited to the strict minimum meaning to one technique, preferably mammography, and if possible to the one view that best imaged the lesion. Ultrasound may be necessary in special cases.

Subsequent examination is primarily concerned with scaring and deformities which each technique must take into account:

- If the excision is extensive the nipple may be off center.
- The scar causes skin folding and possible thickening.
- Postoperative fibrosis may take on a stellate appearance. Nodules can develop either by fibrosis or ductal sclerosis, forming small cysts.
- Microcalcifications may develop if the talc is not completely removed by the surgeon.
- The thermogram is altered by the operation and there is no longer any reference.

It is often necessary to do follow-up thermograms every 3 months. Scar images tend to fade, then stabilize.

Radiotherapy (Appendix, Fig. 149)

It is only 2 months after the end of treatment that two processes develop concurrently: edema and hyperthermia on one hand and postradiation sclerosis on the other. The latter can cause late trophic changes, even years after treatment.

Clinical: Does it depend on the competence of the radiotherapist or the particular characteristics of the tissue response? Anything is possible: from having to double-check to make sure which side was treated, to major sclerosis and telangiectasis where the physician regrets not having recommended mastectomy.

Palpation often detects a mass of induration which resolves in patches, making interpretation particularly difficult.

Transillumination: Light rays clearly differentiate edema (translucent) from sclerosis (opaque). Diaphanometry will eventually be able to quantify these findings.

Ultrasonography: The sonographic image of the tissue changes:
- Skin thickening
- Interstitial edema, causing dissociation of connective tissue and ductal elements

Mammography: Edema creates strong, diffuse opacity in the breast and increases the difficulties involved in compression. The bands are dissociated and the skin is thick. Sclerosis tends to increase the density and number of bands which become evident when the edema diminishes.

Thermography: After treatment a "thermal tide" or diffuse hyperthermia of the treated areas, often reaching 3°–5°C, develops. This hyperthermia usually decreases beginning with the 3rd month after the end of treatment. In some cases, however, it is persistent and may last for more than 1 year. Telangiectases, which usually develop at later stages, cause lower, more localized but definitive hyperthermia.

Stewart and Treves' Sarcoma: Lymphangiosarcoma

This unique lesion develops in the edematous arm on the treated side. Both the radical mastectomy and intense irradiation can be equally implicated. It appears as if a combination of the two is more often the cause and that careful precautions during axillary irradiation considerably reduce the incidence. This may be a local metastasis from the treated breast cancer or, more likely, sarcomatous transformation of lymphangiomatosis.

Clinical: Edema of the arm becomes warm and painful 5–15 years after treatment. Red spots followed by small nodules then appear.

Prognosis: This disease is always fatal.

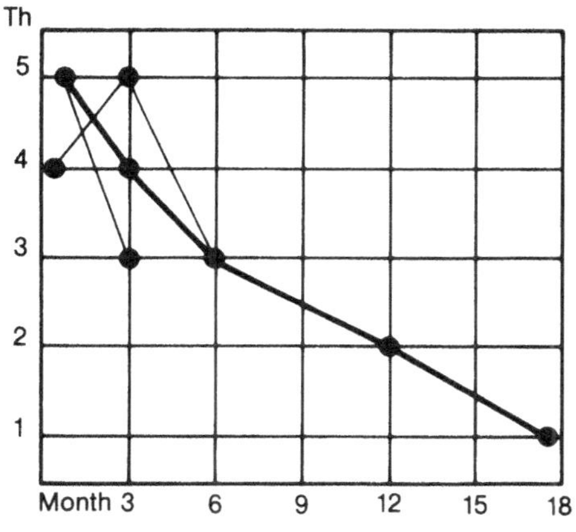

a Progressive linear cooling (Th 5 to Th 2) in one year: sterilization

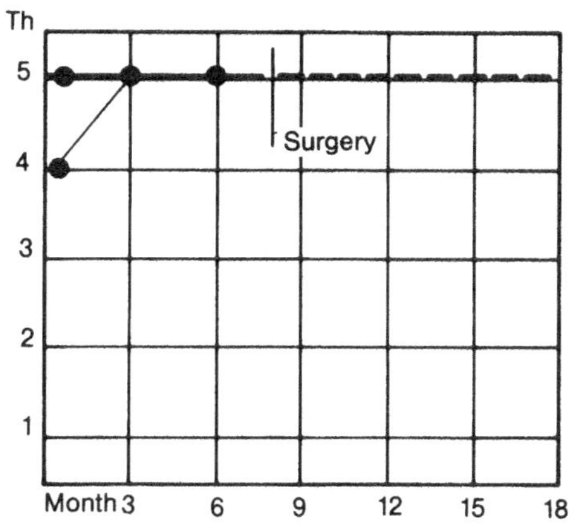

b Persistent hyperthermia at a high level: non-sterilization

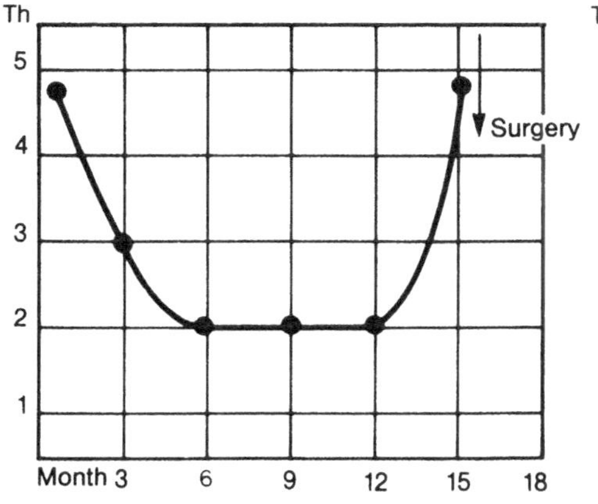

c Image "revives" after transitory extinction, forming a "U" curve (Th 5-Th 2-Th 5): certain recurrence

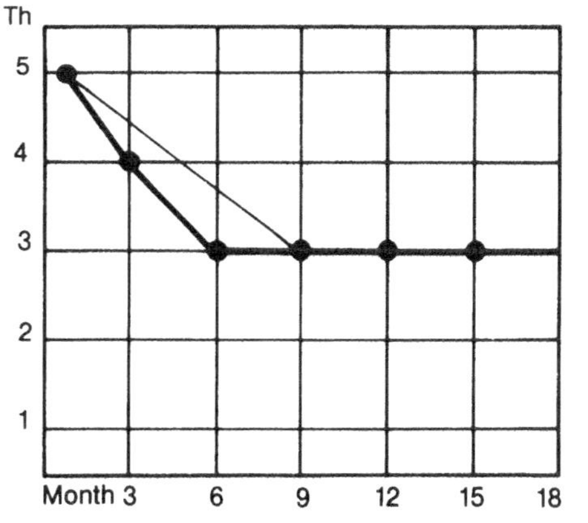

d Hyperthermia persists at an intermediate level (Th 3), with no change after 18 months: radiotherapeutic breast

Fig. 117a–d. The four thermographic courses of breast cancer

Follow-up After Palliative Treatment

A roentgenographic study will determine the effectiveness of treatment 2 months after its completion. Needle biopsy is necessary in the case of colloid carcinoma since the radiographic image persists even after effective treatment. All forms of carcinoma may leave residual opacities due to sclerosis. This is particularly so in the case of scirrhous carcinoma. Close follow-up is essential.

3.5.3.7 Follow-up After Primary Treatment

The patient should be examined every 4 months during the 1st year, postoperatively; then less often until the 5th year, and once a year thereafter. This is to detect any local recurrence as well as any contralateral lesion, of which the risk is greater than 15%. Complete examination is not always necessary. Procedure depends largely on the type of primary lesion. As for telethermography, once the base thermogram is established, repetitive examinations make the detection of any zone of increased temperature particularly significant (Fig. 117).

3.6 Cutaneous and Nipple-Areolar Disease

3.6.1 Benign Florid Papillomatosis of the Nipple (Erosive Adenomatosis of the Nipple)

This occurs between the ages of 28 and 70 years.

Histologic examination is usually necessary to eliminate a diagnosis of Paget's disease.

Papillary formations of ductal cuboidal epithelium develop on the nipple surface. Normally, however, squamous epithelium covers the nipple and lines the terminal ampulla.

There are two possible causes for this condition, both of which probably exist:

- Either actual epithelial ectopy by displacement of the zone separating cuboidal from squamous epithelium. Ulceration develops since the cuboidal cells are less resistant to mechanical irritation.
- Or intraductal adenomatosis spreads to the ductal opening or penetrates under the squamous lining of the nipple and forms a nodule.

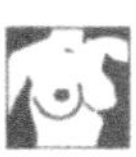

The description is essentially *clinical.* Three appearances can be observed:

1. A nipple nodule without ulceration: pseudotumoral form.
2. A slightly painful, superficial nipple ulceration which weeps or bleeds on contact. The presence of several scabs indicates the need for breast examination and nipple biopsy to rule out Paget's disease.
3. Proliferation of papillary elements at a distance from the ductal opening constitutes the hypertrophic form. The vegitative, granular appearance of the lesion is predominant but superficial ulcerations are also present. These two latter forms represent the actual erosive adenomatosis of the nipple.

Growth

The lesion grows very slowly with remissions that may be long, during which transitory epidermization occurs.

3.6.2 Subareolar Abscess

Even though its clinical expression is due to an infectious process, we discuss it here because of its pathogenesis. This involves ectopy of the epithelium but unlike nipple papillomatosis, here the reverse is true. Squamous cells extend into the duct beyond the lactiferous sinus. Keratinous disquamation causes dilation and obstruction of the duct, leading to local superinfection and formation of a small abscess. A nipple-areolar fistula drains the abscess (Fig. 118). Some authors implicate the involvement of accessory lactiferous ducts.

Clinical: The presenting sign is a purulent discharge from a small opening at the base of the nipple.

Fistula opacification: Since the ductal obstruction is usually incomplete, it is generally easy to show the involvement of the duct either by galactography or by fistula opacification.

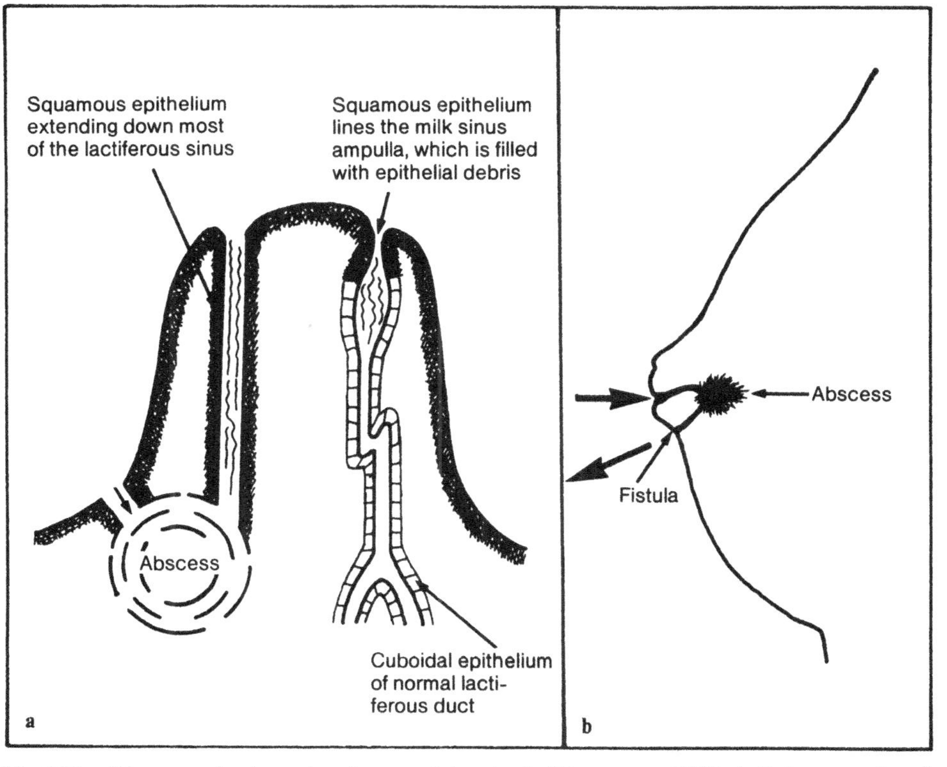

Fig. 118. a Diagram of subareolar abscess of the nipple (Haagensen 1971). **b** Galactography of the subareolar abscess

3.6.3 Sebaceous Cysts

A sebaceous cyst creates a small shadow with transillumination but mammographic interpretation may be more difficult unless the small, round, homogeneous nodular image is viewed tangentially, showing its cutaneous location. More often it appears within the breast. Diagnosis can be difficult when inflammation is involved.

Clinical: The cyst may mimic a subareolar abscess when in the areola (but is usually further from the nipple).

Mammography: The overlying skin appears thickened in a tangential view.

Thermography: The lesion may create a hot zone and presence of the cyst should be carefully noted.

3.6.4 Other Nonspecific Skin Lesions

Naevi, cutaneous fibroma, neurofibromatosis

Each one of these can be detected during inspection and does not require breast examination. However, if undetected, they may, like the sebaceous cyst, be responsible primarily for mammographic errors. They create dense, homogeneous, well-delineated opacities. They are rarely viewed tangentially and are usually seen superimposed on breast tissue, making interpretation difficult.

3.6.5 Primary Melanoma of the Breast

As for any other part of the body, skin covering the breast can be the site of malignant melanoma. Other than its preference for the areola (nipple excluded) it has no unusual sign or symptom. Thermography plays an important role here. It is highly sensitive and fairly specific in detecting this malignant process. Axillary lymph node metastases are frequent. The prognosis is poor.

3.7 Vascular Disease

Malignant diseases (see sarcoma) have already been covered. Here, we will discuss vascular abnormalities and the consequences.

3.7.1 Mondor's Disease

This so-called Mondor's disease is more a syndrome than a disease and was described by Flessinger and Mathieu (1922) before Mondor (1939). It is due to superficial thrombosis of veins overlying the chest. Pain can be a presenting symptom.

Clinical: Its appearance is distinctive; a vertical or oblique, lateral thoracic-mammary fold better seen with the patient's arms raised and in the supine position. The indurated vein can be palpated.

Transillumination: The shadow of the superficial vein is clearly seen with low intensity.

Mammography: It is possible, under good conditions, to distinguish the fine opaque line of the affected vein. Tangential views should show skin thickening and retraction and the absence of any underlying lesion.

3.7.2 Breast Infarction

Embolic obstruction of a breast artery is rare. It does occur in arteritic patients.
- Limited infarction affects the retroareolar region and presents with pain and bloody discharge. It gradually resolves accompanied by periods of local inflammation.
- Massive infarction causing necrosis of a large portion of the breast and even the skin is rare. The cause is unknown.
- It occurs primarily during pregnancy or lactation. Sudden tumoral proliferation or anticoagulant treatment may play a role.

3.7.3 **Hematoma** (Appendix, Figs. 150, 151)

Causes of breast hematoma other than trauma can be attributed to blood anomalies due to anticoagulant treatment or hemopathy. When associated with hematomas in other parts of the body, the cause may be known. Solitary breast hematoma with no known cause should be considered suspect since it may be a first sign of breast cancer.

Clinical: Ecchymosis may accompany the hematoma but clinical signs and symptoms may be absent. Palpation is often negative. Sometimes a firm patch is detected. It takes several weeks, in some cases, for a well-delineated mass to form. This corresponds to cystic transformation of the hematoma.

Transillumination: This is the most distinctive examination: The blood is opaque and creates a clearly distinct shadow.

Ultrasonography: Slight cutaneous thickening is the only finding at an early stage. Later, ultrasonography may show the hemorrhagic cyst. (See "Clinical findings" for a cyst.)

Mammography: The mammographic image may be completely normal since blood has the same radiographic density as the adjacent tissue. Secondary signs may be observed: slight, localized, increase in radiographic density; dissociation of connective tissue bands; skin thickening.

Thermography: No distinctive signs.

3.7.4 **Fat Necrosis** (Appendix, Fig. 152)

This may be caused by local inflammation or occur in older women without known cause. Trauma, however, is frequently involved. (See Sect. 3.8.)

3.8 Breast Trauma

3.8.1 Solitary Closed Trauma

Determination of the actual degree of trauma is subjective on the part of the patient. It may be overestimated in cases of occupational injury, attack, and family quarrel: or minimized when the result of a sports accident, horseplay, or a baby's kick.

In all cases a careful breast examination is in order, and follow-up for at least 1 year. While trauma is generally not considered to have an effect on carcinogenesis, it is not rare that carcinoma be detected during the following year. It may be that the trauma is only a revealing factor or that a preexisting lesion makes the breast more sensitive to even slight trauma.

Signs and symptoms vary considerably from the initial phase: several hours to several days after the trauma, to the cicatricial phase: 3 or 4 months later; different possibilities include: complete remission, formation of a hematoma that may become encysted, fat necrosis (steatonecrosis), causing formation of a fat-encapsulated mass.

Recent Trauma

Clinical: Spontaneous and induced pain is variable as is ecchymosis which may be absent or cover and extend beyond the breast. Palpation is either negative or reveals slight cutaneous edema (thickened skin) or increased localized firmness.

Transillumination: A distinct opacity indicates a hematoma whose size can then be determined.

Ultrasonography: Skin thickening and occasionally edematous skin disassociation are the only findings.

Mammography: Only skin thickening is imaged. A minimum of edema is needed to be seen on the mammogram.

Thermography: There is usually no late change.

Transitory Post-trauma Phase

Clinical: The ecchymosis runs its usual gamut of colors. Any abnormality detected by palpation either disappears completely or leaves a resistant residual nodule.

Transillumination: The shadow of the hematoma decreases and may disappear. The residual nodule can be opaque: encysted hematoma or clear: fat necrosis.

Ultrasonography: Signs of cutaneous thickening and edema diminish. The sonogram may be normal. Two types of images may also appear:
- A cystic lacuna of a hemorrhagic cyst.
- A round lacuna containing few echoes corresponding to fat necrosis.

Mammography: Signs of cutaneous thickening and edema diminish. The mammogram may be normal or three different images may be seen:
- Sclerous, sometimes stellate images.
- A homogeneous nodular opacity of a hemorrhagic cyst.
- The image of fat necrosis: well contrasted, clear and round in an opaque breast or schematically represented in a fatty breast. It is often joined to the skin by several fibrous bands.

Thermography: There is no specific abnormality but fat necrosis can mask an underlying lesion.

Late Post-trauma Phase

- Sclerosis can cause skin and/or nipple retraction.
- The hemorrhagic cyst, whether aspirated or not, disappears, leaving a sclerous stellate image.
- Fat necrosis remains and may calcify.

3.8.2 Microtrauma of the Breast (Bra Syndrome) (Appendix, Fig. 153)

This is due to a poorly adjusted bra. Resulting lesions are minor but should be recognized since they may appear suspect.

Clinical: Pain is the presenting symptom most often involving the submammary fold. The patient usually reports a change in the type of bra, weight gain, or increased breast volume. Palpation of the painful area detects induration and cutaneous edema.

Transillumination: There is no perceptible abnormality.

Mammography: The characteristic image is an opacity corresponding to edema of the submammary fold. It is in the form of a triangle pointing down with overlying thickening and slight retraction.

Ultrasonography and Thermography Are Not Useful

Course: Since certain images are difficult to interpret, a second examination is usually done in 3–4 months.
- When the cause has been eliminated, clinical and radiographic signs disappear.
- Otherwise, fibrous bands and occasionally fat necrosis develop.

These lesions may later calcify. When multiple points are involved, many small rounded dense opacities can be imaged corresponding to Leborgne's calcified microcystic fat necrosis.

3.8.3 Surgical Trauma and Breast Injury

Only nonspecific changes, regardless of the type of operation, are discussed here. We will cover each of the processes involved.

1. *Edema* develops immediately and resolves in several days to several weeks.

2. *Hematoma* can also be detected immediately after trauma – especially with transillumination – and either resolves or forms a hemorrhagic cyst in several weeks to several months.

3. *Fat necrosis* develops slowly and much later. It may be 1 year after surgery before detection. Calcification is frequent.

4. *Sclerosis* is particularly significant since tissue has been sectioned. Fibrous bands can be found in all lengths, thicknesses, and directions. Unfortunately, they frequently converge and often form many stellate images. This sclerosis can also cause formation of small retentional cysts due to ductal obstruction.

5. *Post-trauma calcification* is polymorphic: microcalcifications of sclerous tissue; calcification of a common or hematic cyst and fat necrosis; multiple calcifications of calcified microcystic fat necrosis.

3.8.4 Foreign Bodies

There are two rare cases: the accident involving a needle fragment or thorn, and the deliberate action involving a needle in prison or psychiatric settings. More often the foreign body is postsurgical: needle fragment, drain, compress.

Mammography: This technique makes it possible to directly view the object even if low in density like a wood chip or even a compress. Diagnostic problems may arise due to the local edematous, granulomatous, then fibrous reactions which complicate the radiographic image and can mimic or mask a neoplastic organic lesion.

3.9 The Surgical Breast (Other Than Cancer Treatment)

Nonspecific tissue changes were discussed in the previous section. Changes with specific operations are covered here.

3.9.1 Resections

3.9.1.1 Open Biopsy

All depends on the amount of tissue removed. Results range from the imperceptible to significant deformity with displacement of the nipple as when biopsy extends beyond the quadrant excision.

3.9.1.2 Extracapsular Mastectomy

This is done for certain severe mastoses containing a high degree of displasia which constitutes a local high-risk factor. Usually most of the glandular tissue has disappeared and the breast appears as an empty pocket. The esthetic results are fair in two cases:

- Either because there is a relatively large amount of subcutaneous fatty tissue – which is better.
- Or because the surgery was incomplete. In this case, breast examination (essentially mammography) is important since the risk of cancer for any remaining glandular tissue is significant.

3.9.1.3 Reduction Mammoplasty

Changes in mammary tissue after this type of surgery are usually significant and cannot be classified. Glandular tissue is heterogeneous on palpation and with transillumination, ultrasound, and mammography. There is usually a high degree of tissue change during the 1st year which is often disquieting, especially since it occurs in a highly glandular tissue.

3.9.2 Plastic Surgery Not Affecting the Gland

3.9.2.1 Treatment for Nipple Inversion

This is usually due to short central lactiferous ducts. After galactography, the surgeon sections these ducts.

3.9.2.2 Suspension Mammoplasty

This is done either separately or in conjunction with reduction mammoplasty. Excision of a variable portion of skin is involved and the type of scar depends on the technique.

3.9.3 Augmentation Mammoplasty

Adipose tissue is rarely used. Most often a preformed implant containing silicone or inflated with saline solution is inserted. The incision is either circumareolar or submammary.

The prosthesis is placed either between the pectoral muscle and the breast or posterior to the muscle.

Clinical: One of the surgeon's goals is, in a sense, to make the clinical diagnosis of his efforts difficult. Fortunately, glaring scars are rare. The breasts have a more homogeneous consistency when palpated.

Transillumination: The retromammary space is clear.

Ultrasonography: Sonograms of the implant clearly demonstrate the sonolucent nature of the fluid and show its outline.

Mammography: The image of silicone is homogeneous and moderately dense. The contour of the implant is distinctly seen due to the tangent effect.

Complications

Sclerosis may thicken the capsule around the prosthesis. This can be palpated and causes peripheral induration. Mammography shows the globular deformity of the implant. Treatment involves excision of the capsule. Occasionally part of the prosthesis folds or the valve of an inflatable can be felt. When diagnosis is difficult, it is for the surgeon to determine procedure since an attempt at needle biopsy may have disastrous consequences.

3.10 Mastitis

Different causes can be implicated in inflammatory breast syndromes:
- Microbial invasion, in specific conditions (post-partum, wound, sting, or bite), of a normal breast; or with preexisting abnormalities (ductal ectasia, cyst, galactocele)
- Tissue intoxication by products of significant catabolism
- Carcinoma

In this first section we will cover general features of acute mastitis. Symptoms are strongest during this phase but provide few specific elements to help determine the cause.

How the disease progresses and its response to treatment will help to make this diagnosis. Benign signs should be considered suspect until inflammatory carcinoma can be formally ruled out. Secondly, then, we will discuss the different clinical courses of acute mastitis according to cause and, finally, primary chronic mastitis.

3.10.1 Acute Mastitis (Appendix, Fig. 154)

The purpose of the examination is:
- To confirm the inflammation
- To determine the type of extension
- To determine the cause

3.10.1.1 Confirming the Mastitis

The inflammatory syndrome involves the mobilization and local influx of elements of the body's defense by blood and lymph. Vessels are dilated, capillary permeability is increased and intracellular spaces are basic signs of inflammation: pain, redness, mass, and heat.

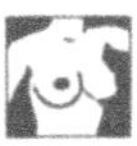

Clinical: The patient will indicate the type, intensity, and site of pain. Inspection will determine the reddish or pink coloration of the skin, which can involve the entire breast, or be localized or along lymphatic pathways. Venous dilation is also noted.

Palpation: Is difficult due to the pain. Skin thickening (with *peau d'orange*) and possibly the underlying mass will be detected.

Transillumination: This may show the opacity of an associated lesion but inflammation itself does not create a shadow.

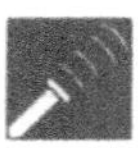

Ultrasonography: This will confirm the cutaneous thickening. It also shows the edematous dissociation of the breast tissue.

Mammography: This should be gently carried out due to the pain and tenderness of the breast. It also demonstrates and determines the degree of skin thickening. Subcutaneous fatty tissue is compressed due to swelling of the underlying tissues and its density increases. There is a diffuse, poorly delineated decrease in translucency corresponding to the inflammatory zone. Its intensity varies depending on the surrounding tissue since this is an aqueous opacity which appears distinct in adipose tissue but is barely perceptible in already dense tissue.

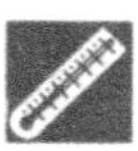

Thermography: Increased vascularization and fairly extensive hyperthermia of variable intensity.

3.10.1.2 Determining the Type of Extension

Paramastitis

Inflammation not involving the glandular tissue in early stages.

Cutaneous and Subcutaneous Lymphangitis (Supramastitis) (Fig. 119)

Clinical: Red bands on the skin, toward the axilla, correspond to lymphatics. The skin is very thick. Painful axillary adenopathy is frequent.

Ultrasonography and mammography: The skin is highly thickened.

Thermography: Hyperthermia varies in intensity and extent.

Inframastitis (Fig. 120)
This involves the retromammary fat (of Chassaignac). Inflammation may originate in this area but is more likely to have spread from deep mammary lobes.

Clinical: The breast is painful and particularly tender at the periphery. It projects slightly but no mass is palpable. General signs of infection may be detected.

Mammography: The opacity of the lesion is much more distinct when it appears in a clear, fatty zone. This is a diffuse, heterogeneous condensation of the retromammary fat with deep mammary condensation.

Localized (or Lobular) Parenchymatous Mastitis (Fig. 121)

Most of the abnormalities in this case involve the glandular tissue itself and constitute the clinical picture of acute galactophoritis.

Clinical: Signs of inflammation are restricted to one sector, quadrant, or two quadrants. Usual signs and symptoms occur in the corresponding areas: pain, erythema, mass with skin thickening and heat – all of which develop suddenly.

Mammography: The signs described above are localized. Sometimes condensation in the involved area is outlined by the relative translucency of the surrounding tissue.

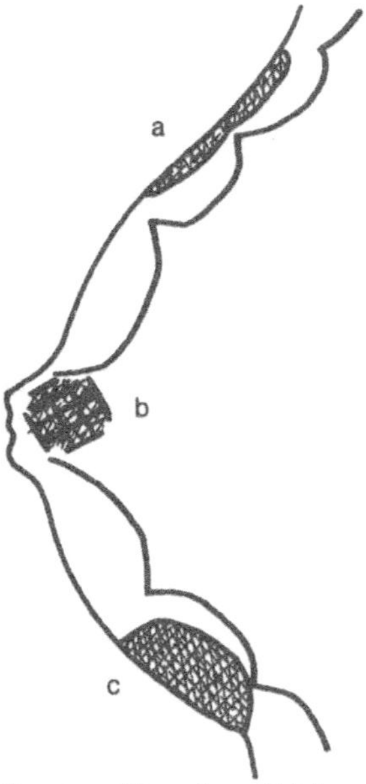

Fig. 119. Supramastitis. **a** Superficial lymphangitis; **b** retroareolar abscess; **c** abscess of lymphangitis

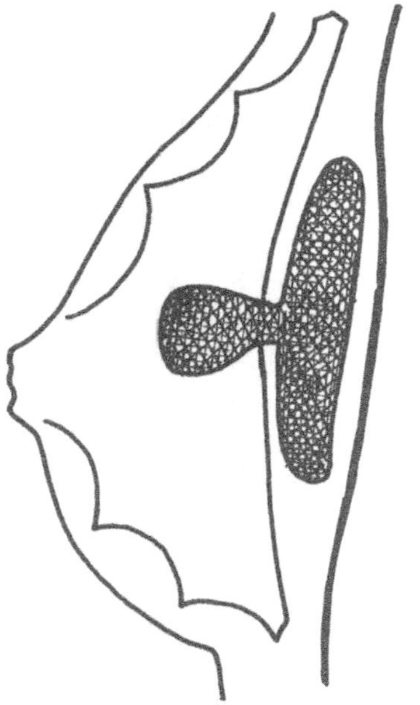

Fig. 120. Inframastitis. Originates in the retromammary area. Possible extension to the parenchyma

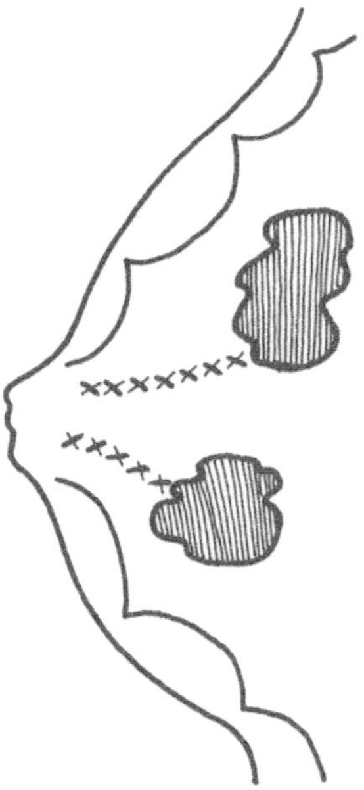

Fig. 121. Localized parenchymatous mastitis

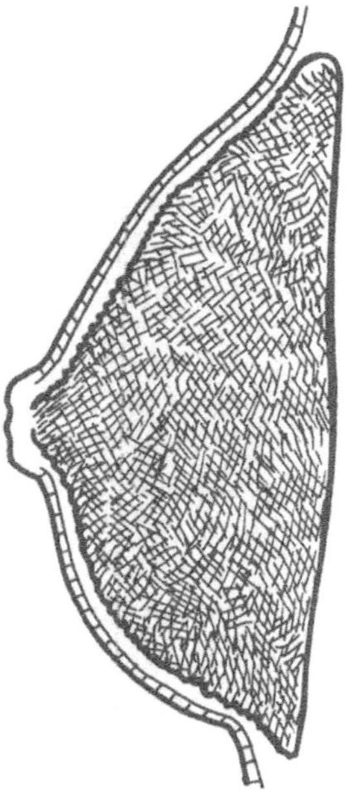

Fig. 122. Panmastitis

Thermography: Hyperthermia is localized or at least predominant in the involved area.

Acute Panmastitis (Fig. 122)

The clinical picture is striking: Signs of inflammation are at their maximum intensity and extent.

Clinical: The breast is painful, red, swollen, and very warm. Its skin is stretched and shiny; veins are dilated.

Ultrasonography and mammography: These examinations are made difficult by the pain and edema. Each shows significant skin thickening and diffuse, edematous infiltration of the glandular as well as subcutaneous adipose tissues.

Thermography: Distinct, massive hyperthermia of several degrees extends beyond the breast.

3.10.1.3 Determining the Cause of Mastitis

Signs of inflammation are in no way specific. Other examination findings and the context are used to help determine the cause. Inflammatory carcinoma is the main preoccupation.

Acute Infectious Mastitis

- Puerperal mastitis develops specifically during postpartum and in a specialized medical and paramedical setting which helps to make the diagnosis and correctly treat the infection. All types can develop, from lymphangitis to panmastitis.
- Diagnosis of superinfection of a cyst, galactocele, or ductal ectasia is obviously facilitated by prior knowledge of the lesion.
- Other causes include wounds, trauma, and bites or stings.

Acute Tubercular Mastitis

This is rare, polymorphic and difficult to diagnose – especially in the acute form. It may be caused by transmission from a cold abscess through the retromammary fat or develop within the breast. The cause is usually only suspected when diagnosis of tuberculosis of another organ has already been made.

Plasma-Cell Mastitis

This recurring infection occurs from menopause on, in women who have nursed. It is considered to be due to concentrated secretions within the ducts which cannot be excreted either because connective tissue fibrosis reduces ductal permeability or the secretions are too thick. The inflammatory reaction includes an influx of plasmacytes; hence the name.

Symptoms are those of a lobular, generally para- or retroareolar mastitis with several characteristic signs.

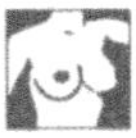

Clinical: The nipple can be retracted and the skin is pink. There is a slightly tender underlying mass and local edema causes skin thickening with *peau d'orange;* a thick, mono- or multiductal discharge is often detected.

Mammography: Other than the typical signs of localized mastitis, the mammogram may show the sinuous, ribbon-like shadow of a large congested lactiferous duct. If the ductal congestion is old, intraductal calcifications may be detected: large oval or rod-like calcifications 1–2 mm long. One extremity is sometimes split corresponding to a ductal division.

Prognosis: Excellent, but diagnosis is sometimes very difficult – especially in pseudotumoral forms.

Involution Mastitis

The distinction between plasma-cell and involution mastitis is a theoretical one as far as classification goes. This really should not be a problem for the physician in his everyday practice. It is important to recognize, however, that this is a distinctly different process. Inflammation is not caused by intraductal congestion but excessive production or insufficient elimination of products of cellular catabolism within the tissues. It may, then, occur during all phases of breast involution, particularly in young women.

Inflammation is rarely intense and can affect a localized area or the entire volume of both breasts. It resolves spontaneously in several days; if not, the diagnosis must be systematically questioned.

Carcinomatous Mastitis or Inflammatory Carcinoma (see Sect. 3.5)

There is no clear limit between the clinical and paraclinical signs of metabolic hyperactivity accompaning invasive carcinoma and the clinical picture of panmastitis caused by massive invasion of dermal lymphatics by cancerous cells. Diagnosis is not a problem if presence of the carcinoma is already known or if it demonstrates characteristic symptoms in addition to signs of inflammation. Otherwise, since inflammatory symptoms lack specificity the physician should always have in mind the possibility of carcinoma when confronted with signs of inflammation and no known cause.

3.10.1.4 The Course of Acute Mastitis

Regression

If the inflammation is quickly treated, symptoms regress without sequelae. It is a good rule to do a complete examination to detect the responsible lesion once the breast becomes supple and painless again.

Abscess (Appendix, Fig. 155)

Abscess formation is the rule when mastitis is due to infection of a cavity: cyst, galactocele, ductal ectasia. It may also occur in normal tissue. The type of mastitis will determine its site but symptoms are similar for all abscesses.
- Lymphangitis causes subcutaneous abscesses.
- Inframastitis causes abscesses in the retromammary fat.
- Parenchymatous mastitis causes solitary or multiple glandular abscesses.

Clinical: the symptoms of mastitis begin to regress and can be found concentrated in one area, where a poorly delineated, sometimes resistant, painful mass can be palpated.

Transillumination: The abscess is opaque.

Ultrasonography: The abscess is well demonstrated by this technique. It presents as a fairly well delineated lacuna with thick, absorbant walls. Several unevenly distributed echoes appear in the lacuna. They correspond to necrotic debris. The beam is reinforced but less so than for a cyst.

Mammography: The appearance differs depending on the stage of development. The diffuse shadow of mastitis fairly rapidly gives way to the homogeneous opacity of the abscess. As inflammation and edema regress, the contour of the abscess becomes more distinct.

Thermography: Changes in the thermogram follow the course of the lesion: attenuation and localization of the hyperthermia.

Chronic Mastitis

3.10.2 Chronic Infectious Mastitis

Whether it follows an acute phase or begins as a low-grade infection, ruling out carcinoma is often difficult. Actually, this partial regression of inflammatory signs or their low-grade appearance is very similar to signs of carcinoma. This type of infection is extremely polymorphic and only rarely does one observe a characteristic clinical picture of nonpurulent subacute mastitis.

Clinical: The skin is variably colored, infiltrated, and retracted.

Transillumination: The involved zone is opaque.

Mammography: The mammogram shows a stellate opacity with bands extending to the skin, which is retracted and thickened.

As one can see, even this form is not reassuring since it has a number of features in common with the scirrhus. Unless other decisive elements are demonstrated, cytologic or histologic examination should make the diagnosis.

3.10.3 Subacute and Chronic Tuberculosis, Cold Abscess

As polymorphic as it is rare, breast tuberculosis is infrequently diagnosed without cytologic or histologic examination. Only a known concurrent TB infection will evoke the diagnosis. The acute form was considered above. As does a common infection, tuberculosis may have a nonspecific chronic clinical picture. This diffuse form frequently has many of the same symptoms as the scirrhus and inevitably leads to histologic diagnosis after biopsy. The cold abscess either forms directly or is transmitted from the chest wall. It can be solitary or multiple and has symptoms typical of a common infectious abscess. Inflammatory symptoms are very slight, however, and the clinical picture is more suggestive of pseudotumors with a differential diagnosis of cysts. Diagnosis of breast TB is based on histologic examination after biopsy or slide analysis of a ductal discharge which sometimes occurs. It is best if the diagnosis of tuberculosis is being considered when studying these fluids.

3.10.4 Mycosis and Parasitosis

This is a section on rare breast diseases.

3.10.4.1 Actinomycosis

Painful mass suggestive of an abscess or carcinoma. Diagnosis may be based on the study of a discharge with characteristic yellow granulations.

3.10.4.2 Echinococcal Infestation

A hydatid cyst of the breast will have mass type symptoms.

3.10.4.3 Filariasis

Diagnosis is relatively easy when the microfilaria are calcified: 2- to 3-cm-long coiled, sinuous filaments. Other localizations of this parasitosis and the etiologic context help to make the diagnosis.

4 Examination Procedure

It is important to define the procedure. The examination should be carried out according to the desired goal. If all could accept this principle, arguments concerning the value of the different techniques could be resolved.

Four procedures can be outlined:

1. Cancer screening
2. Examination and diagnosis of a breast disease
3. Follow-up of a treated or untreated breast disease
4. Diagnosis of breast cancer

These are the basic areas of concern and obviously any unexpected discovery must be thoroughly investigated.

4.1 Cancer Screening

Cancer detection is something all physicians are concerned about but we consider here the problem of mass screening. This can be done on two levels: screening for the risk of cancer and actual cancer detection.

4.1.1 Risk of Cancer

Earlier we considered the principle risk factors. The importance of one factor alone should not be exaggerated. Several factors together, however, may lead to a thorough examination and special follow-up, where the least symptom is taken into consideration. The risk related to certain mastosis with epithelial proliferation should be recognized. Mammograms could be used to establish this risk but such a method is not problem-free. In addition, it requires systematic mammography, which is a major initial examination. Diaphanometry, as we have seen, may eventually provide an easy noninvasive method for screening these particular risk factors.

4.1.2 Carcinoma

Statistics in the United States (where the incidence is slightly higher than in western Europe) show that 5% of women will some day develop breast cancer.

Considering the advantage of early treatment, screening asymptomatic women makes sense. Different techniques have been used. The value of each is based not only on its reliability (sensitivity and specificity) but also on cost, ease, and time involved in using the equipment.

4.1.2.1 Telethermography

This technique was primarily used for the ease with which it could be handled in mass screenings. Too good to be true, it was disappointing. Its specificity is only passable since it demonstrates the hyperthermia of simple inflammation or endocrine disorders. Its sensitivity is particularly poor when it comes to detecting a quiescent lesion – particularly in situ carcinoma, which is generally cold. Thus, this was one of the reasons for which a technique as valuable as thermography was so severly criticized by serious specialists. Let us make a comparison. What physician making a diagnosis of acute appendicitis would be negligent in obtaining a rectal temperature? Undoubtedly, none. Yet if a screening for appendicitis were to be organized, certainly no one would base it on rectal temperatures.

4.1.2.2 Ultrasonography

This is an analytic type technique. To examine both breasts fully, even with an automatic unit, would take more time than would be feasible for simple screening.

4.1.2.3 Mammography

There is no doubt that, for women over 50 years of age, this is the best method for screening in light of its sensitivity as well as its specificity. Unfortunately, it is relatively costly and high in irradiation.

We will not be the last to point out that this irradiation is weak, especially with the use of rare earth screens, and that no serious study has been able to attribute any increased incidence in cancer to it. Nevertheless, it has yet to be proven completely harmless and this must be a prerequisite for any systematic examination to be repeated once a year.

4.1.2.4 The Clinical Examination

Screening based on a clinical examination, particularly palpation, is fairly inexpensive, noninvasive, and easily repeated. In addition, its performance is quite respectable, at least in France where the effort to inform the public about the importance of regular breast examination has not always had the anticipated response. Without a need for organizing special screenings, regular breast examination by the family physician (each woman is examined by a physician an average of 2.6 times per year) as well as the occupational physician plays a valuable part in detection. By regularly performing this examination, each physician, by his acquired competence, can considerably increase its effectiveness.

4.2 Examination and Diagnosis of a Breast Disease

This is the most common breast examination procedure: a symptom indicates a need to detect an abnormality:

- Functional?
- Benign organic:
  Localized?
  Multifocal?
  Diffuse?
- Malignant?
- Associated with a lesion of another nature?

With what we currently know, all possible means available must be used to uncover and study all information. There is no valid reason to ignore or detract from this conception of breast examination. It is not essential to do everything the same day or in the same place. Nevertheless, this is the best way to coordinate the different techniques and make the most of their interpretation. The time saved goes without saying.

The order in which the different techniques are used is not arbitrary:

1. Interview (may be done during thermographic cooling)
2. Thermography
3. Clinical examination
4. Transillumination
5. Ultrasonography
6. Puncture-insufflation: for cysts
7. Mammography (cystography when appropriate)
8. Needle biopsy for solid nodules as required
9. Analysis

Using this order makes it possible to avoid unnecessary mammography prior to puncture-insufflation of cysts. It is desirable, but unfortunately not always possible, to obtain results of the needle biopsy before analyzing the data. Usually the analysis must take into consideration different possibilities depending on the pathology report and, consequently, even different possible decisions. This is important since often the physician who obtains the biopsy is the best suited to interpret the value and weaknesses of a negative result in each case.

4.3 Follow-up of a Breast Disease

It may be malignant or benign, treated or untreated. It may also refer to an unexplained symptom. Follow-up examination make it possible to make comparisons over a period of time. The schedule of visits and type of examination are extremely variable from one case to the next. Comparison of two examinations performed at different times is valid only if each item has its proper reference in order to verify that a change is not due to altered technical conditions. This is especially true for thermography, where it is necessary to consider the appearance of areas other than the breast and for mammography where overall blackening must be the same for both films.

4.4 Diagnosis of Cancer

Absolute proof of carcinoma either by cytologic or histologic examination is necessary before the therapist can begin anticancer treatment. Both require localization of the lesion, and palpation is by far the most accurate. Localization of nonpalpable lesions, be they radiographic or sonographic, is difficult and tedious. This special objective of the therapist owes its high success rate to the classic "triad": palpation, to determine where it is; mammography, to verify it exists; and needle aspiration, to see if it is cancerous. Once the diagnosis is confirmed, it is up to the therapist to make a thorough study of the cancerous disease:

- Local examination: size, site, extension, histologic type, and hormone receptors
- Breast examination: condition of the tissues, detection of a distant, ipsi- or contralateral lesion
- Regional examination: adenopathy
- General examination:
  Metastases
  Immunology
  Biological markers

It is also important to regroup local elements in order to determine a prognosis: clinical (TNM, PEV), thermographic (Q class), cytologic, or histologic (cytoprognosis, grade).

5 Analysis

Analysis will vary depending on the type of examination.

5.1 Detection

Whatever the technique used, there are two possible conclusions:
- Negative
- Need for further examination

It is not desirable at this point to determine specificity of the results or distinguish between benign and malignant disease. In this way, one avoids making a haphazard diagnosis with insufficient data. This will also ease the situation for the people concerned.

5.2 Diagnosis of Cancer

The pathologist's report provides the answer. Except in rare cases, it is a yes or a no with indications as to the histologic type and degree of invasion.

5.3 Cancer Work-up

This involves bringing together the elements necessary for establishing a treatment procedure or for estimating the results of treatment. This is where the therapist takes over or, at least, intervenes in choosing the necessary examinations.

5.4 Final Analysis

This is where the conclusion should be thoroughly established. It involves transforming a collection of sometimes conflicting data from diverse examination

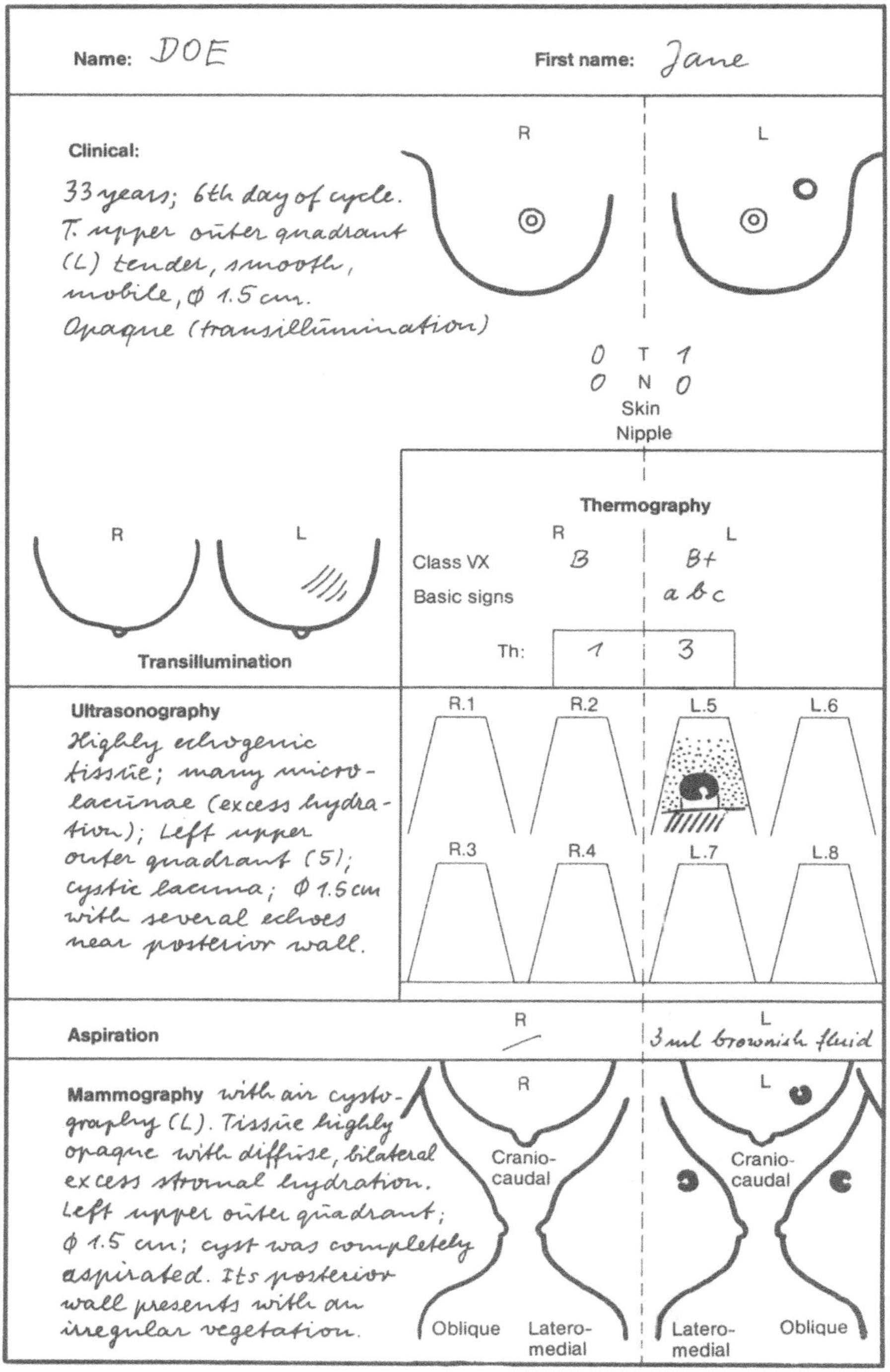

Fig. 123. Data from the various examination techniques

Table 6. Interpretation of data in Fig. 123 and suggested plan

12 September 1985

Mrs. Jane Doe

Breast examination requested by Dr. Smith

Mass in left breast suddenly appeared 10 days ago

Functional examination
- Signs of excessive glandular stroma hydration

Organic examination
- The mass proved to be a cyst which underwent puncture-insufflation
- The posterior wall presents with an irregular vegetation

Screening factors
- Precocious puberty
- Late first pregnancy

Suggested plan
- Open biopsy
- Medical treatment to reduce the excess hydration

techniques into a coherent conclusion with two, sometimes, overlapping, parts (Fig. 123).

1. The answer to the problem that required the examination
2. The report of the breast cancer screening: identification of high-risk factors; detection of an asymptomatic lesion

The results are divided into four sections (Table 6):
- Functional examination
- Organic examination
- Screening factors
- Suggested plan

5.4.1 Functional Examination

With an acceptable approximation, the intensity of estrogenic hyperactivity is determined according to the degree of stromal hydration and that of overall hormonal hyperactivity according to signs of lobular proliferation (transillumination densification, nodular mammogram, lobulations seen with ultrasonography). Despite its subjective nature it may be of help to the therapist in making a choice. Any galactorrhea is included in this functional examination.

5.4.2 Organic Examination

5.4.2.1 Types of Breast Tissue

1. Variations of normal tissue: overall degree, fibrous tendency, degree of fatty tissue
2. Mastosic tissue: proliferating, cystic, fibrous

Transillumination, ultrasonography, and mammography provide the necessary findings to determine the above.

5.4.2.2 Is There a Lesion?

The combined results offer three possibilities:
1. No abnormality was detected.
2. A lesion was clearly detected with no conflicting evidence. For example: easily palpated nodule, distinct radiographic image, well-delineated lacuna. No further examination is needed for confirmation.
3. There is some doubt. In a difficult-to-study breast with dense tissues, one or several techniques show a zone where the tissue appears altered:
   - Palpation: increased firmness
   - Transillumination: slightly opaque patch
   - Ultrasonography: a less echogenic zone or an area with several small lacunae but no distinct contour
   - Mammography: increased opacity

   Here the physician has two alternatives:
- Thermography: a warm spot in the questionable zone is indication for immediate cytologic if not histologic examination.
- Follow-up after medical treatment (hormone, anti-inflammatory, or vascular). Persistence of the abnormality, even if isolated, after 2–3 months should also lead to cytologic or histologic examination.

5.4.2.3 Is the Lesion Malignant?

The Lesion is Palpable and Well Delineated

This is the easiest situation since needle biopsy can be immediately obtained. If interpretation is difficult open biopsy will provide the answer.

The Lesion is Palpable and Poorly Delineated

Other techniques may demonstrate high suspicion of carcoma in which case open biopsy is immediately obtained. They may also be negative. This is often the case of a lesion in a mastosic patch. Its firmness and stability are cause for concern. Needle biopsy may be judged too arbitrary and open biopsy too severe. Here again, thermography or follow-up 2–3 months after treatment will help to decide in favor of open biopsy.

The Lesion Is Not Palpable

- The technique that detects it indicates a high probability of malignancy.
- Ultrasonography: lacuna with a strip of absorption; mammography: scirrhus or spiculated nodule. A nonpalpable lesion often can be palpated once the physician is alerted to its existence. In this case, it falls into the above category. A truly nonpalpable lesion poses the problem of its localization.

Sonographic localization is impractical with an immersion unit since the prone position and unsupported breasts make needle insertion virtually impossible.

Automatic transducers make localization much easier. The most precise localization, however, is achieved with manual transducers. It is important to obtain a significant A mode image. A mode transducers specially adapted for needle insertion do exist but are not frequently used.

Mammographic localization: A simple procedure makes use of a metallic grid during compression. The grid is left in place and serves as a reference point during biopsy. A Swedish method of spatial localization using needles, with the patient in the prone position, is more precise but requires more complex equipment.

5.4.3 Screening Factors

These are risk factors; but the word "risk" has an unnecessary, dramatic connotation. The interview will provide the necessary information. Certain factors may influence the diagnosis in that they call for a stricter interpretation of the symptoms. Often they help determine the schedule for follow-up.

5.4.4 Suggested Plan

It is not for the diagnostician to dictate procedure to the therapist. Nevertheless, in light of his examination findings he is in a position to propose certain indications:

- Immediate diagnostic procedure: open biopsy
- Follow-up examination at a specific time following medical treatment to alleviate the consequences of excessive functional activity
- Type of treatment when a functional disease or mastosis is involved

Appendix

Fig. 124. Adipose breast

Fig. 125. Excess hydration

Fig. 126. Adenomas and fibroadenomas

Fig. 127. Phylloide tumor

Fig. 128. Sclerosing adenosis

Fig. 129. Dystrophic cyst

Fig. 130. Lactiferous duct ectasia

Fig. 131. Papillary adenoma

Fig. 132. Oil cyst

Fig. 133. Diffuse mastosis

Fig. 134. Lipoma

Fig. 135. Hamartoma (fibroadenolipoma)

Fig. 136. Comedocarcinoma

Fig. 137. Intraductal papillary carcinoma

Fig. 138. Intracystic papillary carcinoma

Fig. 139. Paget's disease of the nipple

Fig. 140. Scirrhous carcinoma

Fig. 141. Nodular carcinoma

Fig. 142. Diffuse carcinoma

Fig. 143. Inflammatory carcinoma

Fig. 144. Invasive lobular carcinoma

Fig. 145. Medullary carcinoma

Fig. 146. Colloid carcinoma

Fig. 147. Solid sarcoma

Fig. 148. Hemangioendothelioma

Fig. 149. Irradiated breast

Fig. 150. Hematoma

Fig. 151. Hemorrhagic cyst

Fig. 152. Fat necrosis (steatonecrosis)

Fig. 153. Microtrauma

Fig. 154. Acute mastitis

Fig. 155. Abscess

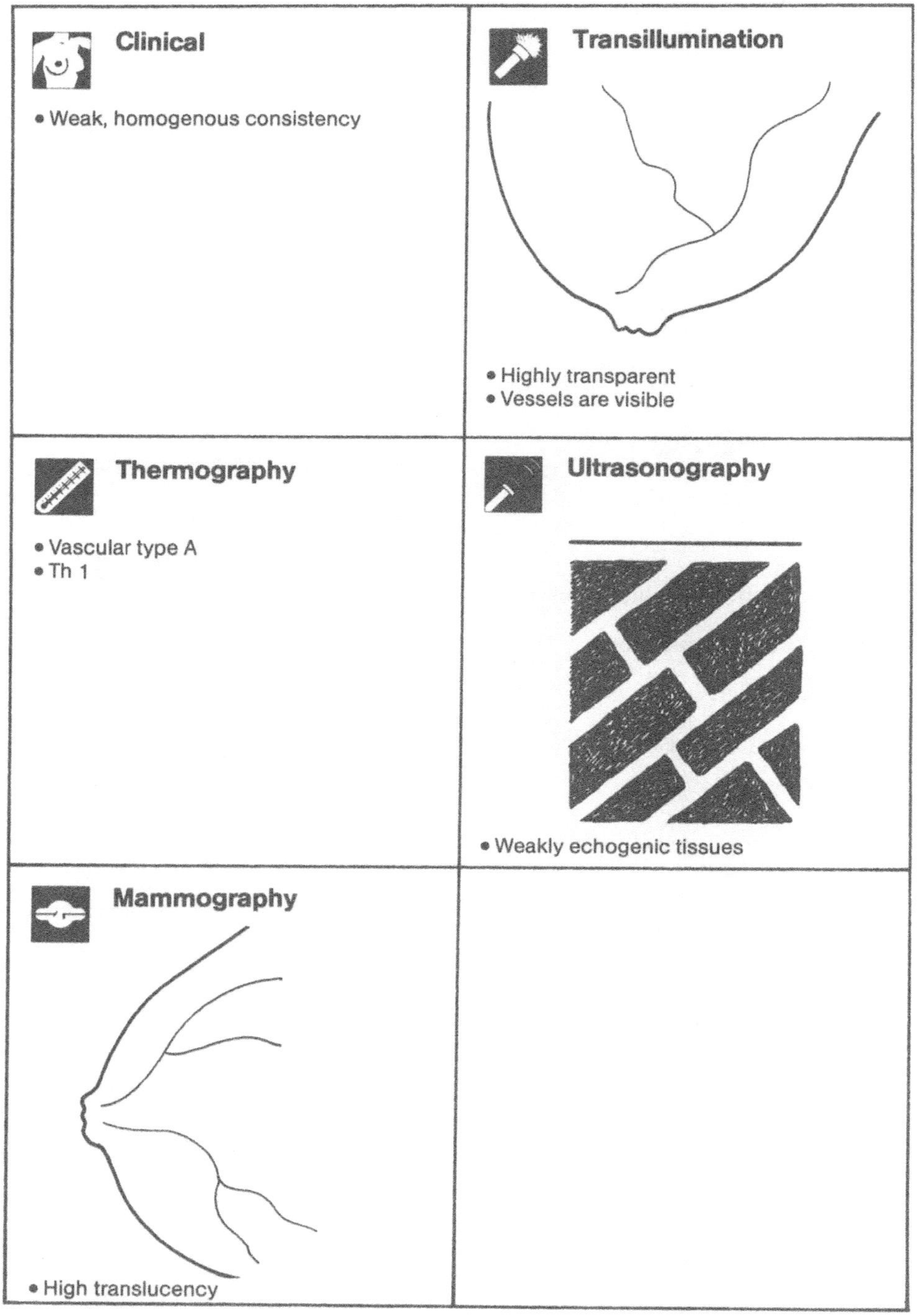

Fig. 124. Adipose breast

Clinical

- Pain
- Firm consistency

Transillumination

- No particular opacity

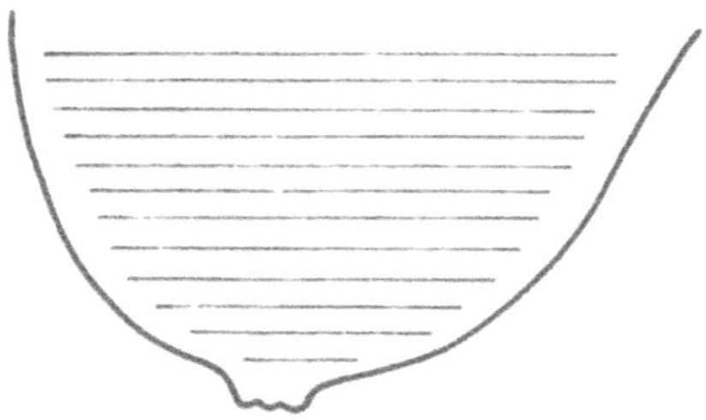

Thermography

- Vascular type B or B+
- Th 2 or 3

Ultrasonography

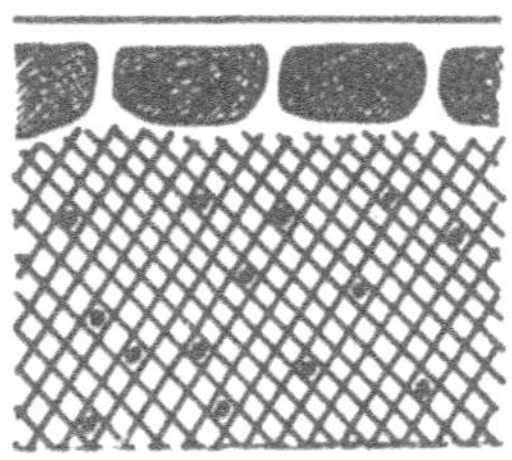

- Tissues accentuated by translucent interstitial edema
- Microlacunae of excess hydration

Mammography

- Highly opaque

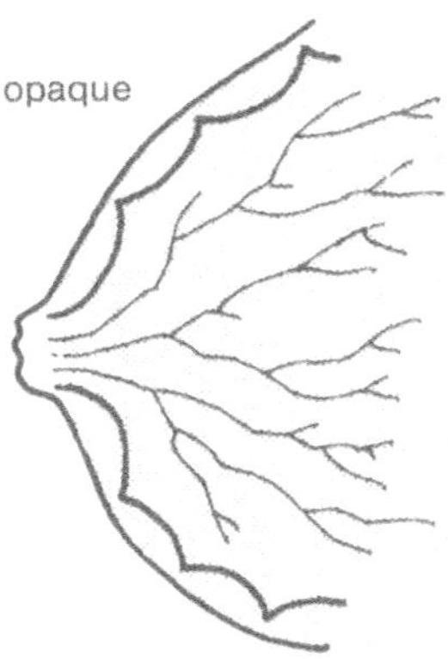

Fig. 125. Excess hydration

Clinical

- Frequent in young girls
- Firm, smooth, mobile mass

Transillumination

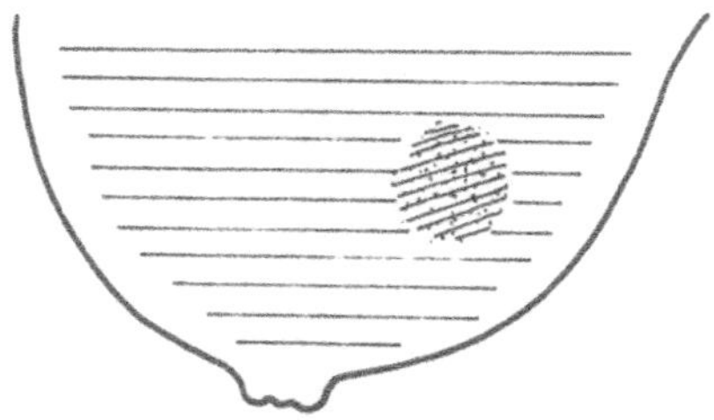

Thermography

- Th 1 or 2
  Giant fibroadenomas:
- Th 3

Ultrasonography

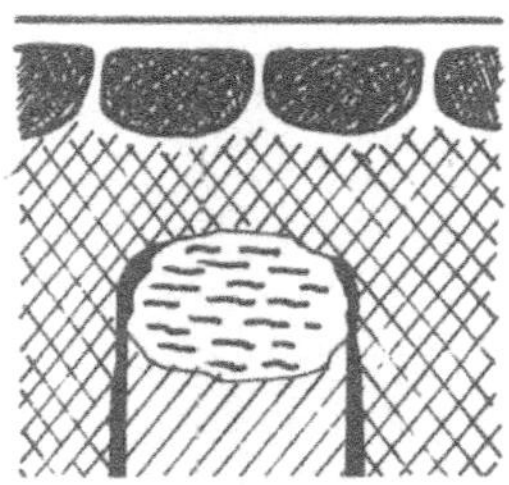

- Distinct lacuna with lateral shadows (except adenomas); evenly distributed echoes

Mammography

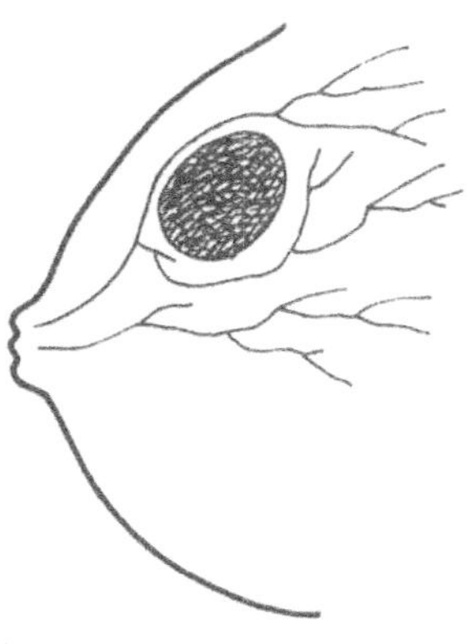

Cytology

- Valid if accurate localization

Fig. 126. Adenomas and fibroadenomas

Clinical

- At puberty and premenopause
- Large mass
- Edema
- Venous network

Transillumination

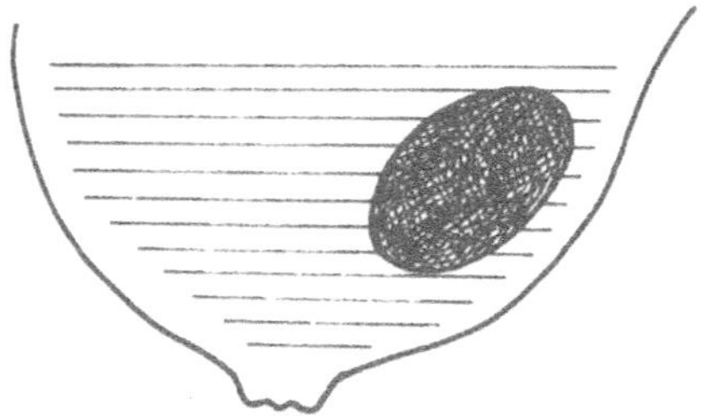

Thermography

- Th ≥ 3

Ultrasonography

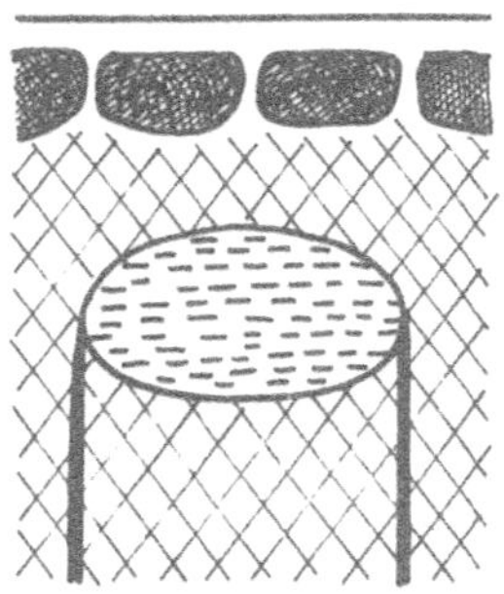

Mammography

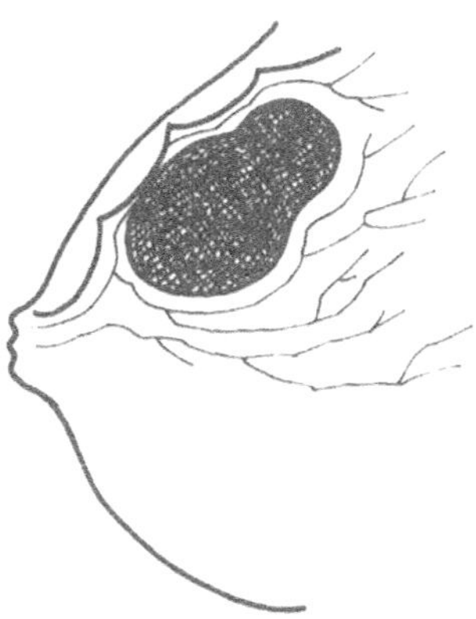

Cytology

- Easy, but excision is required

Fig. 127. Phylloide tumor

Clinical

- Irregular, mobile mass

Transillumination

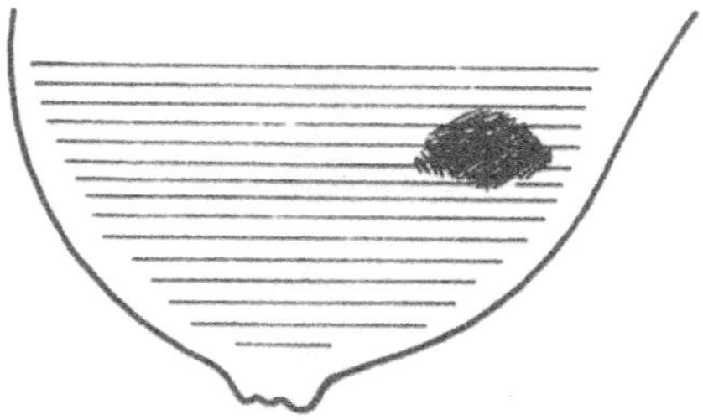

Thermography

- Th 1 or 2

Ultrasonography

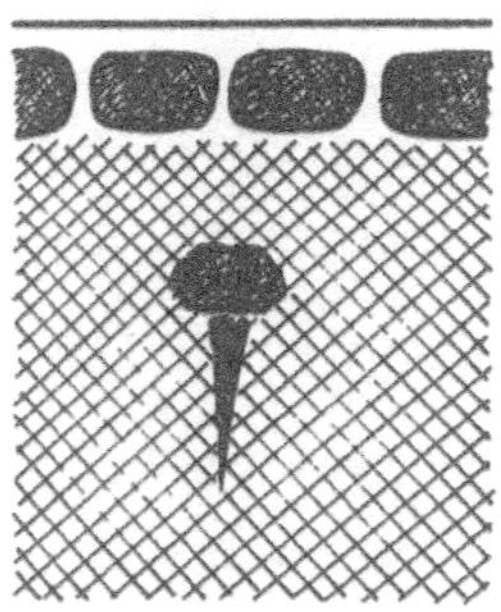

Mammography

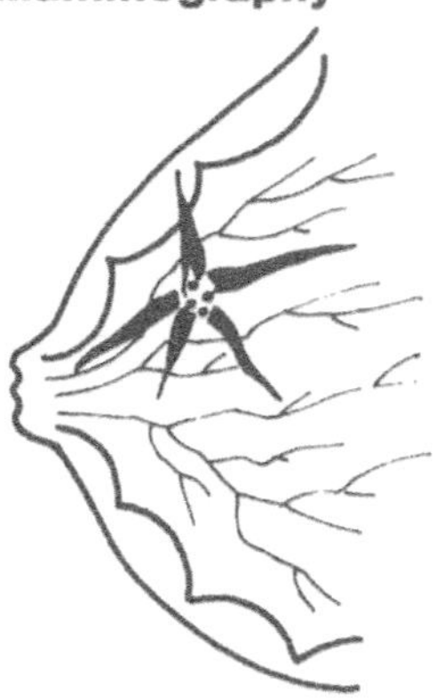

Cytology

- N/A

Fig. 128. Sclerosing adenosis

Clinical

- Sudden appearance of a painful mass
- Firm, smooth, mobile
- Resistant

Transillumination

- Opacity if fluid is dark

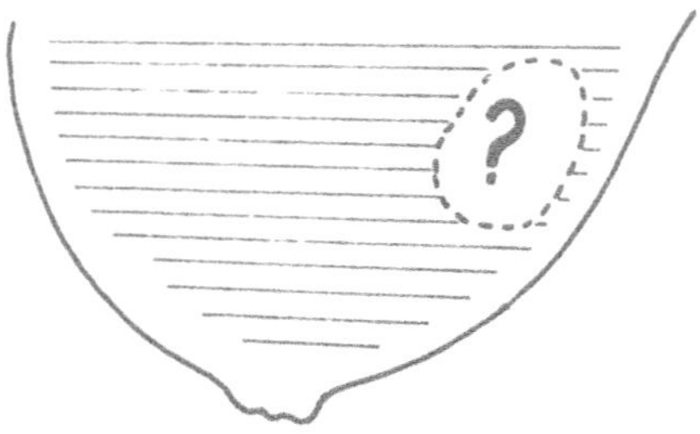

Thermography

- Th 2 or 3

Ultrasonography

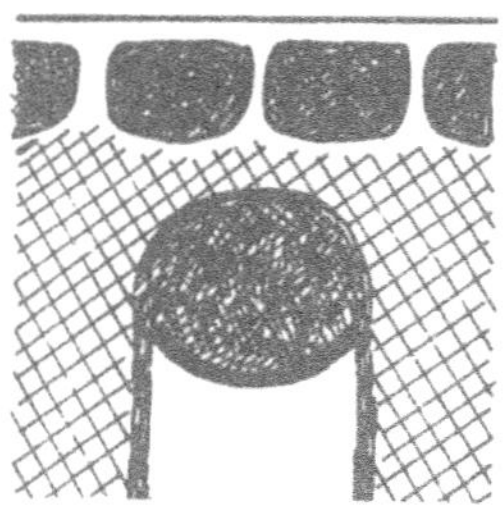

- Fluid lacuna
- After insufflation: absorbant gaseous lacuna

Mammography

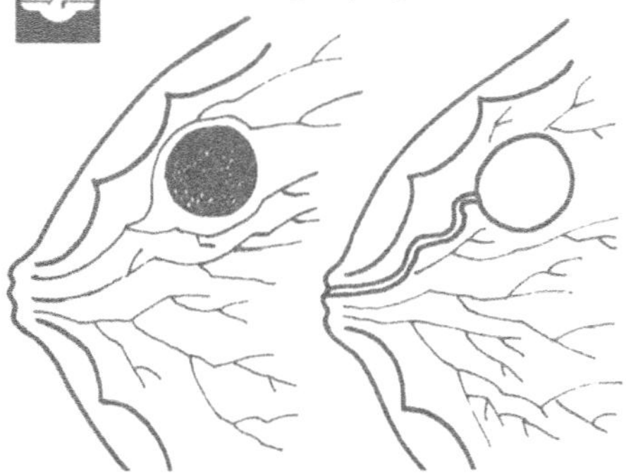

- Insufflation: air transparency; air galactogram

Cytology

- Fluid centrifugation: results are generally not significant

Fig. 129. Dystrophic cyst

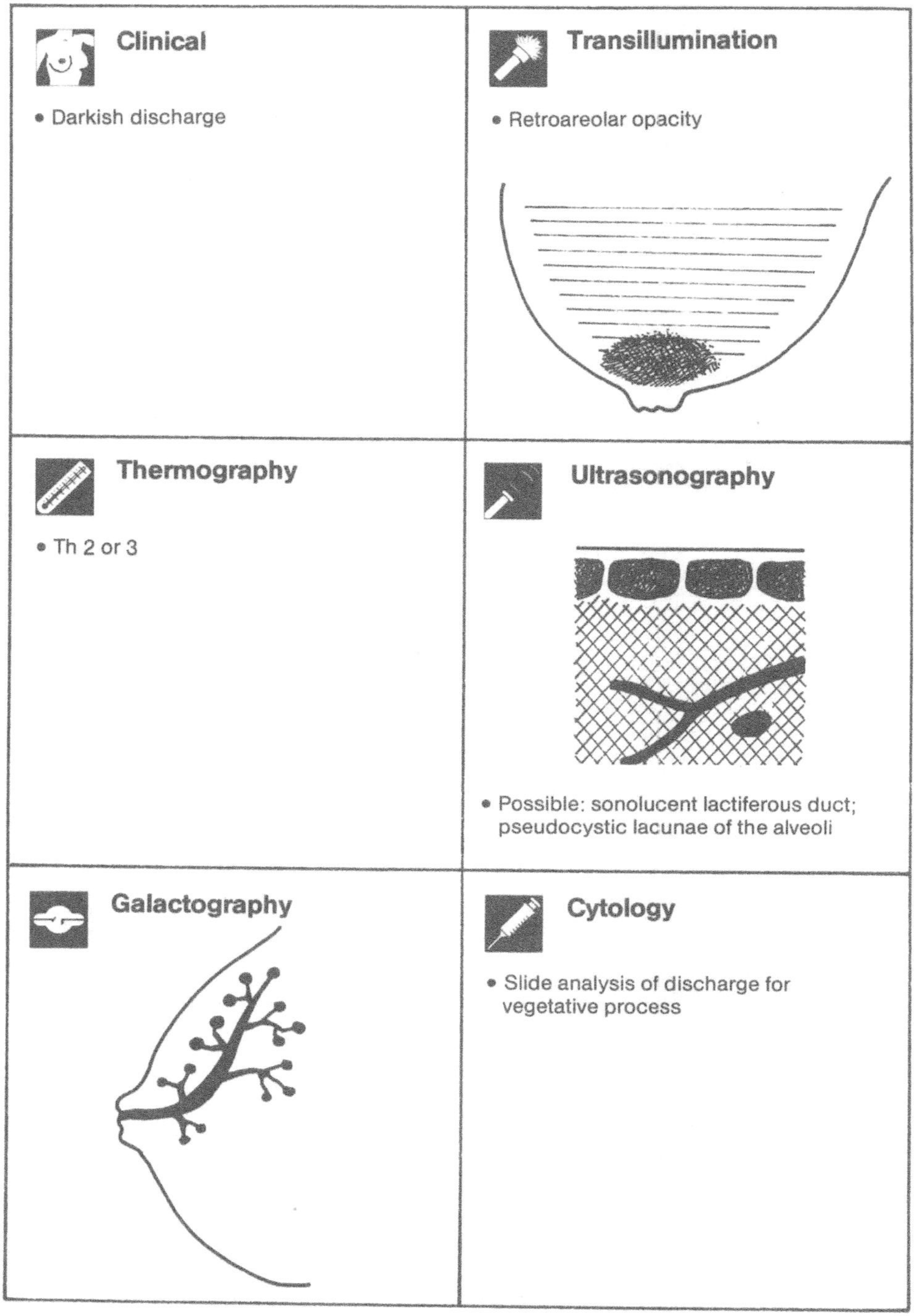

Fig. 130. Lactiferous duct ectasia

Clinical

- Bloody or brownish discharge
- Possible palpable nodule

Transillumination

- Retroareolar opacity; possible opacity of the lesion

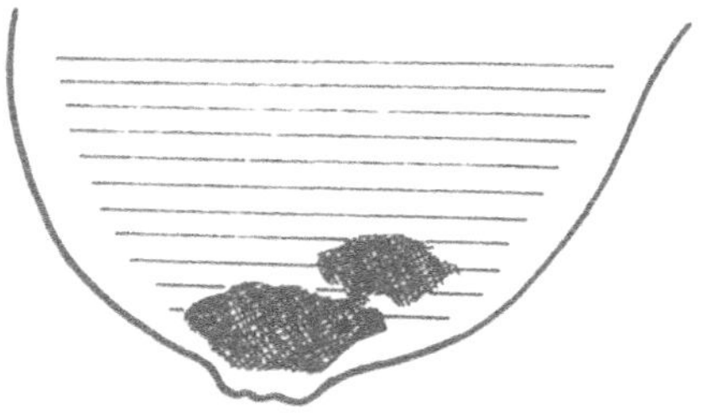

Thermography

- Th 2 or 3

Ultrasonography

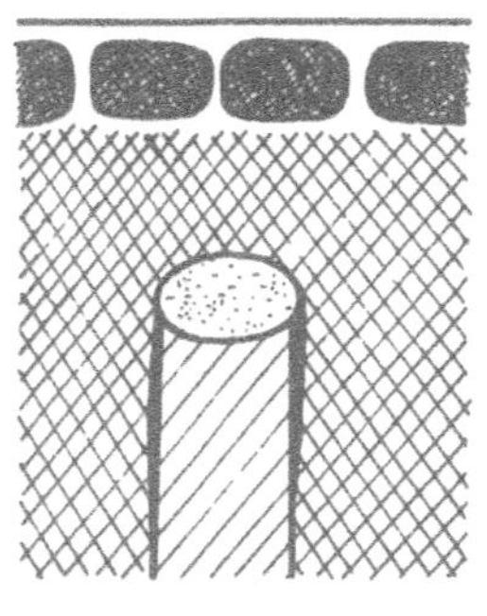

Galactography

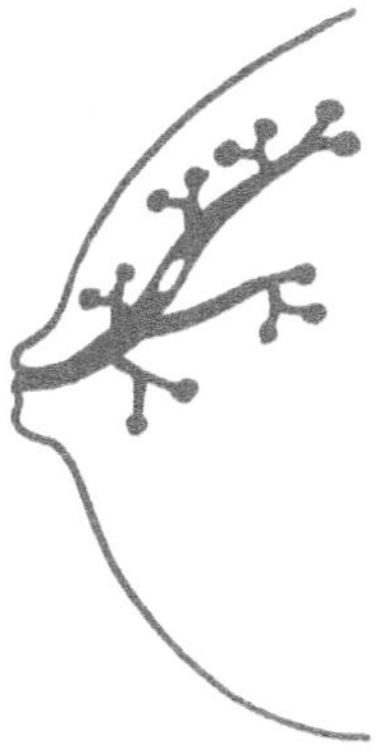

Cytology

- Slide analysis of the discharge: highly suggestive papillary cell masses

Fig. 131. Papillary adenoma

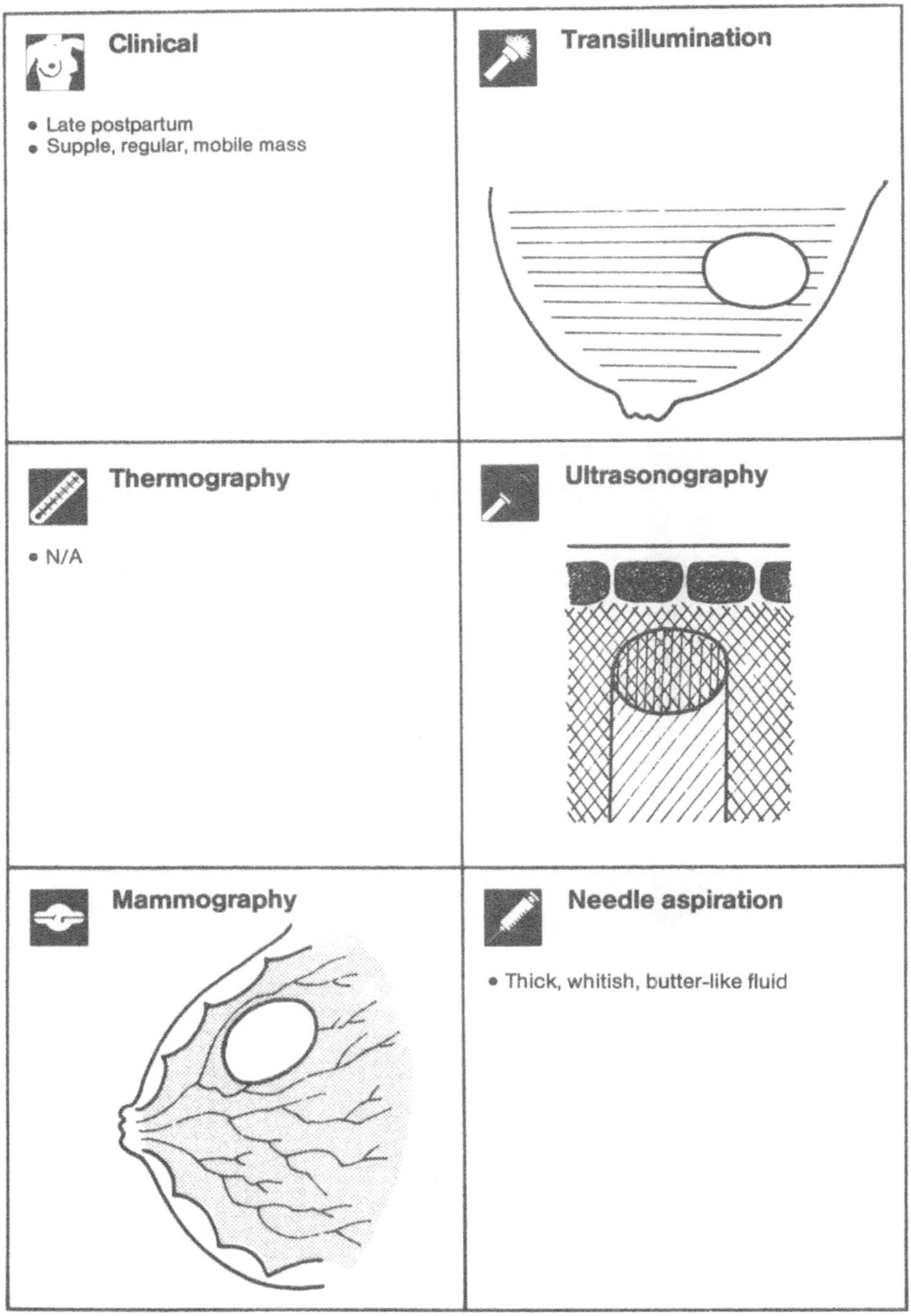

Fig. 132. Oil cyst

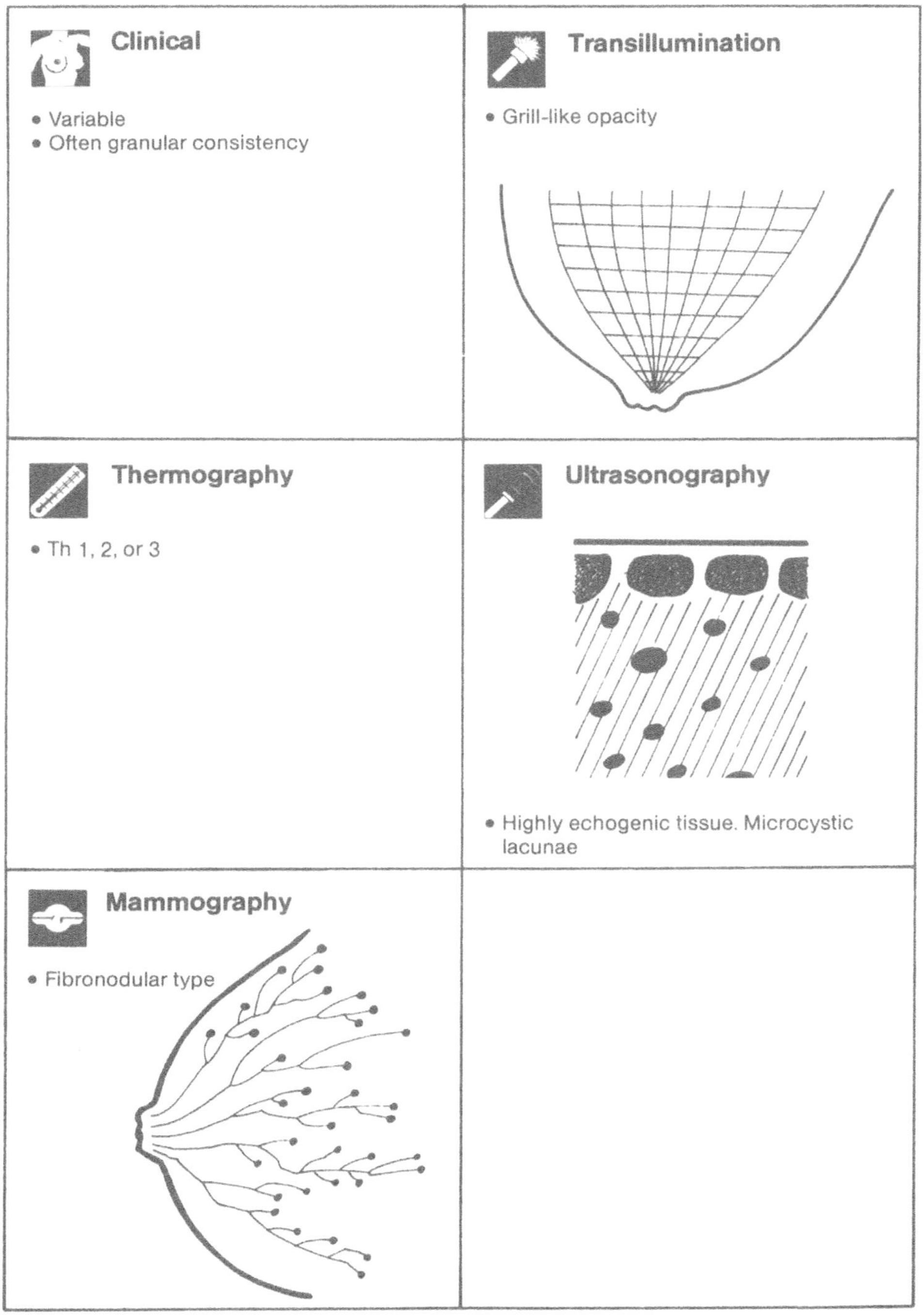

Fig. 133. Diffuse mastosis

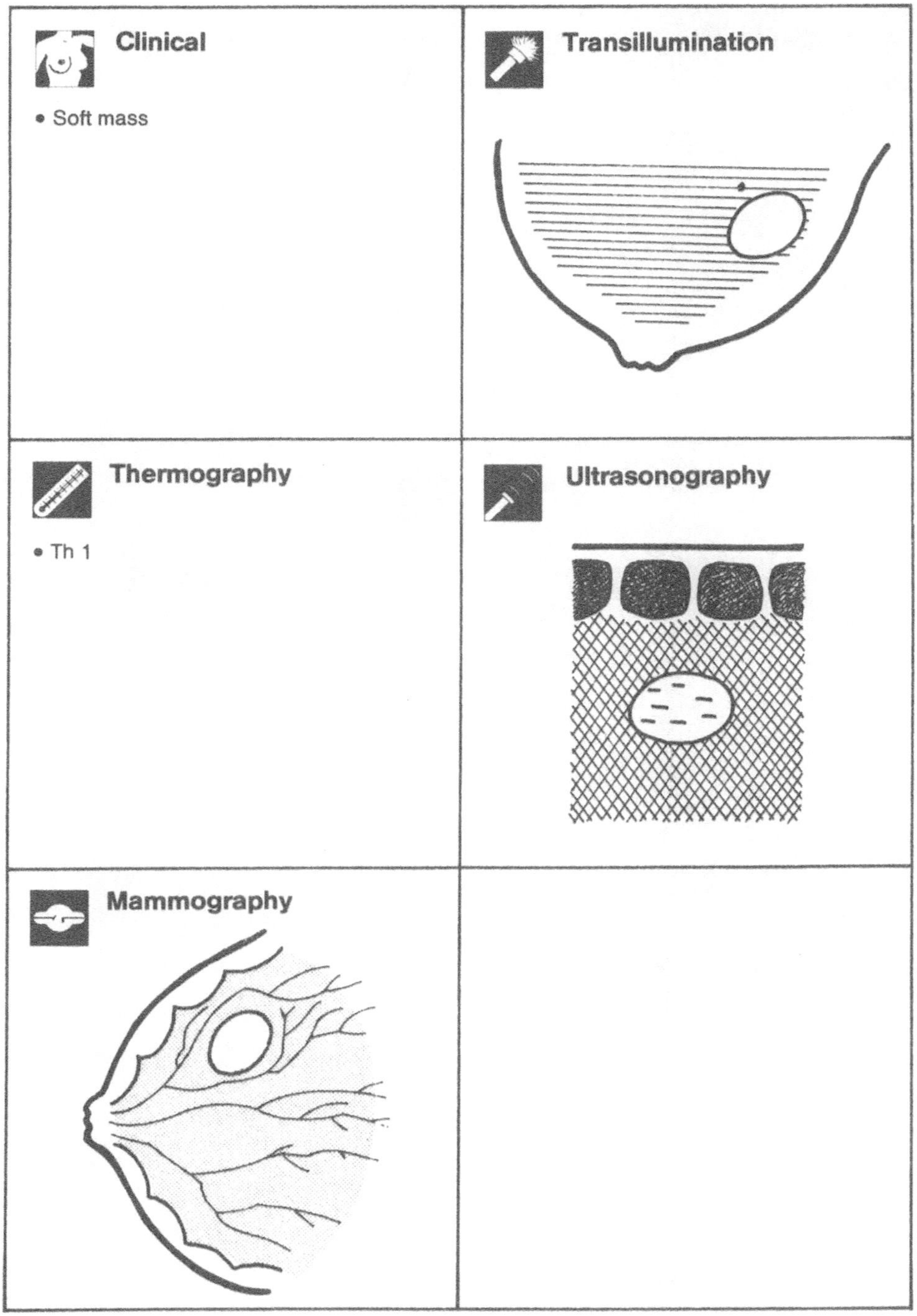

Fig. 134. Lipoma

Clinical

- Well-delineated but malleable mass

Transillumination

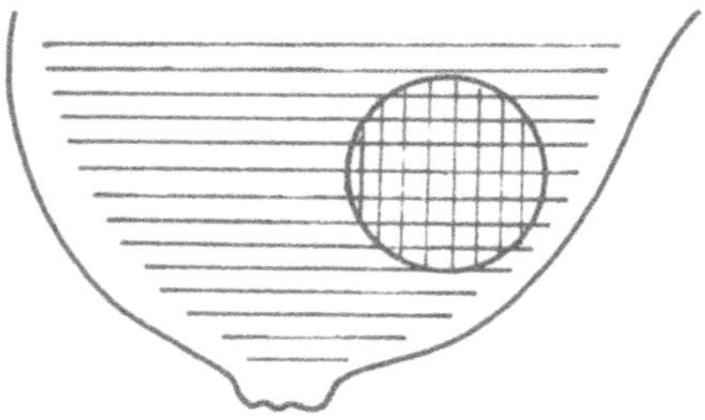

Thermography

- Th 1 or 2

Ultrasonography

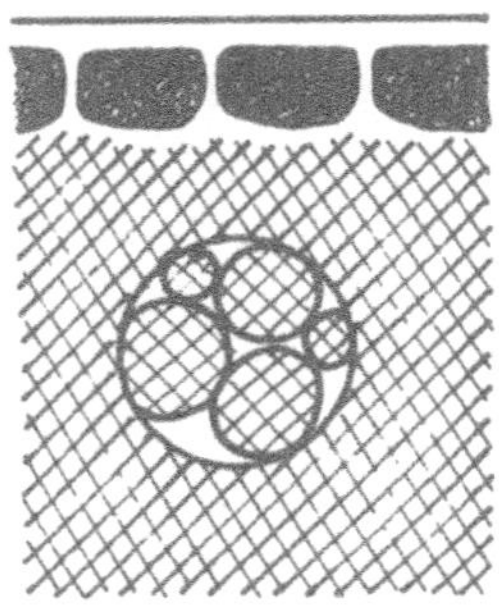

Mammography

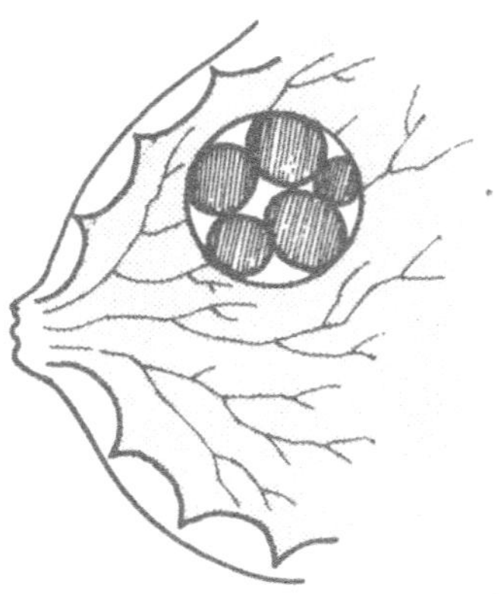

Fig. 135. Hamartoma (fibroadenolipoma)

Clinical

- Diverse signs
  - Discharge
  - Paget's disease of the nipple
  - Localized induration

Transillumination

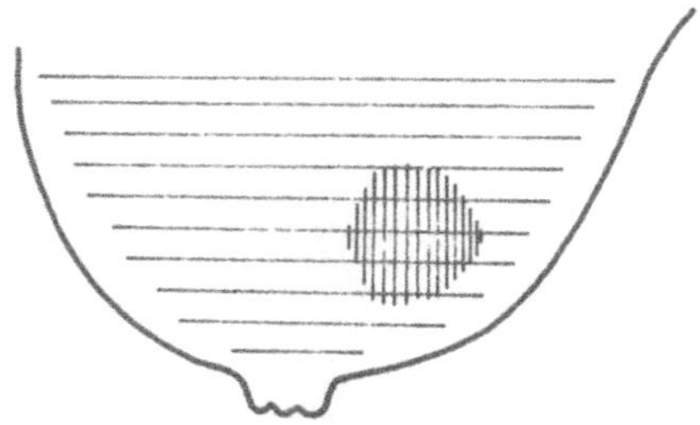

Thermography

- Preinvasive phase: Th 1 or 2
- Invasive phase: Th ≥ 3

Ultrasonography

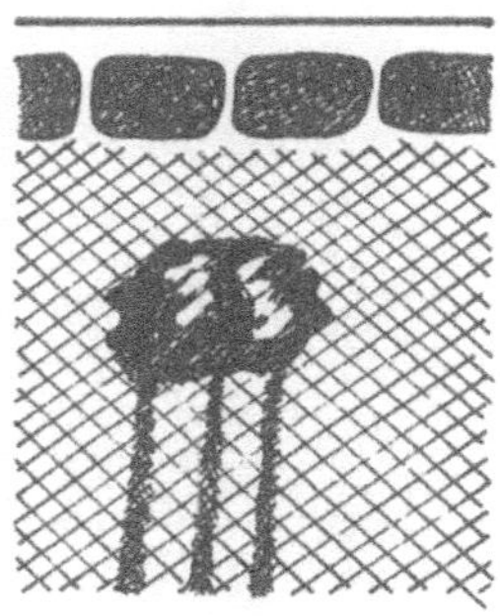

Mammography

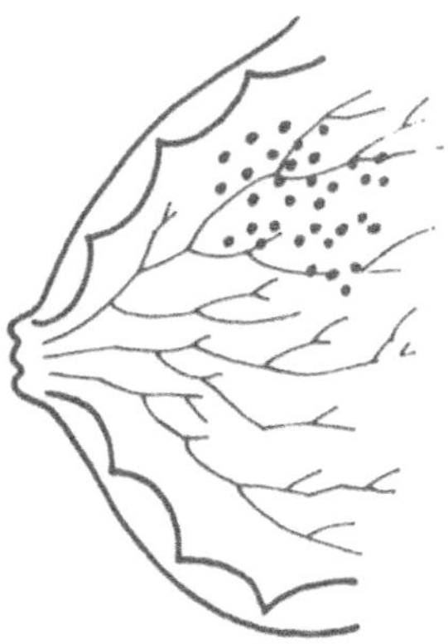

Cytology

- When discharge, slide analysis may make the diagnosis

Fig. 136. Comedocarcinoma

Clinical

- Bloody discharge (pencil sign)

Transillumination

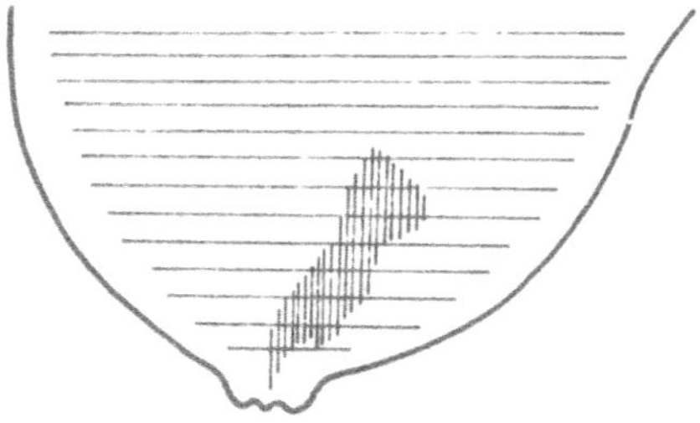

Thermography

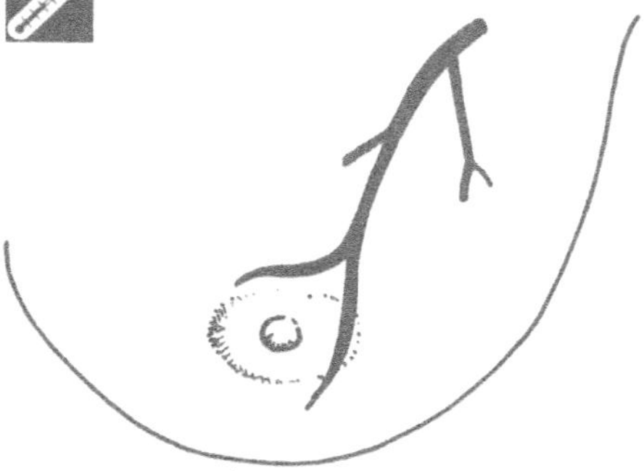

- Preinvasive phase: Th 2
- Invasive phase: Th $\geq$ 3

Ultrasonography

N/A

Mammography

N/A

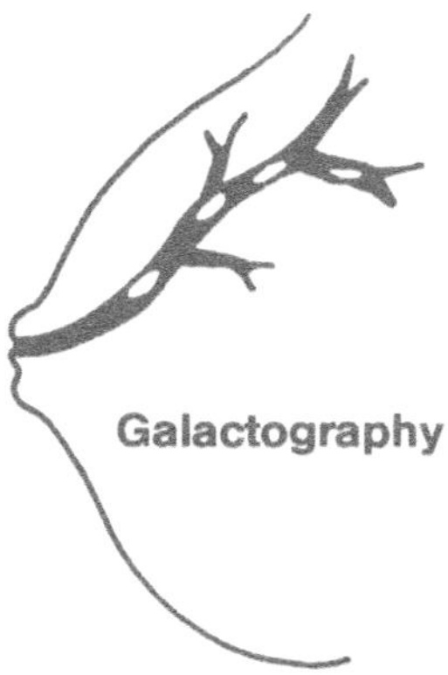

Cytology

- Slide analysis of the discharge may make the diagnosis

Fig. 137. Intraductal papillary carcinoma

Clinical

- After the age of 50 years: sudden appearance of a hard, regular, painful nodule

Transillumination

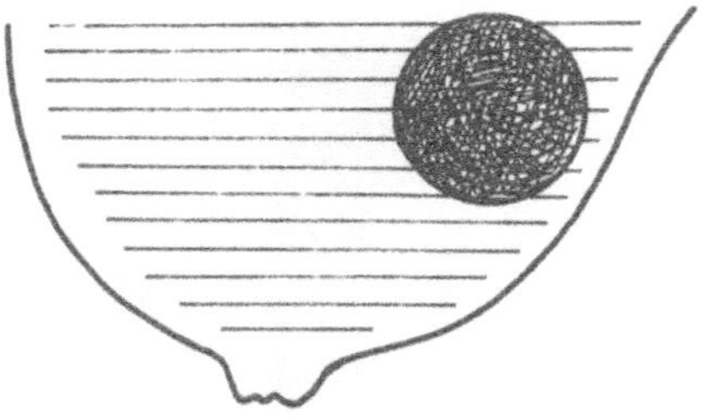

Thermography

- Preinvasive phase: Th 1 or 2
- Invasive phase: Th ≥ 3

Ultrasonography

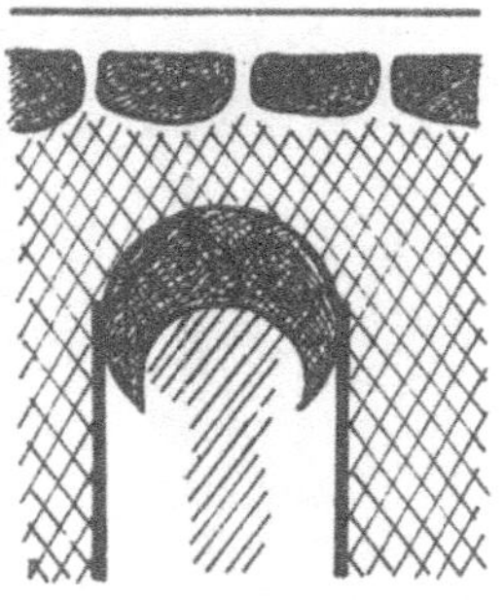

Mammography

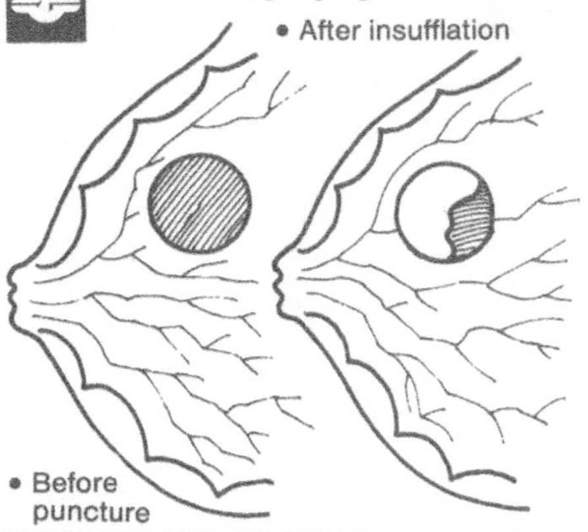

Cytology

- The fluid specimen may provide the diagnosis

Fig. 138. Intracystic papillary carcinoma

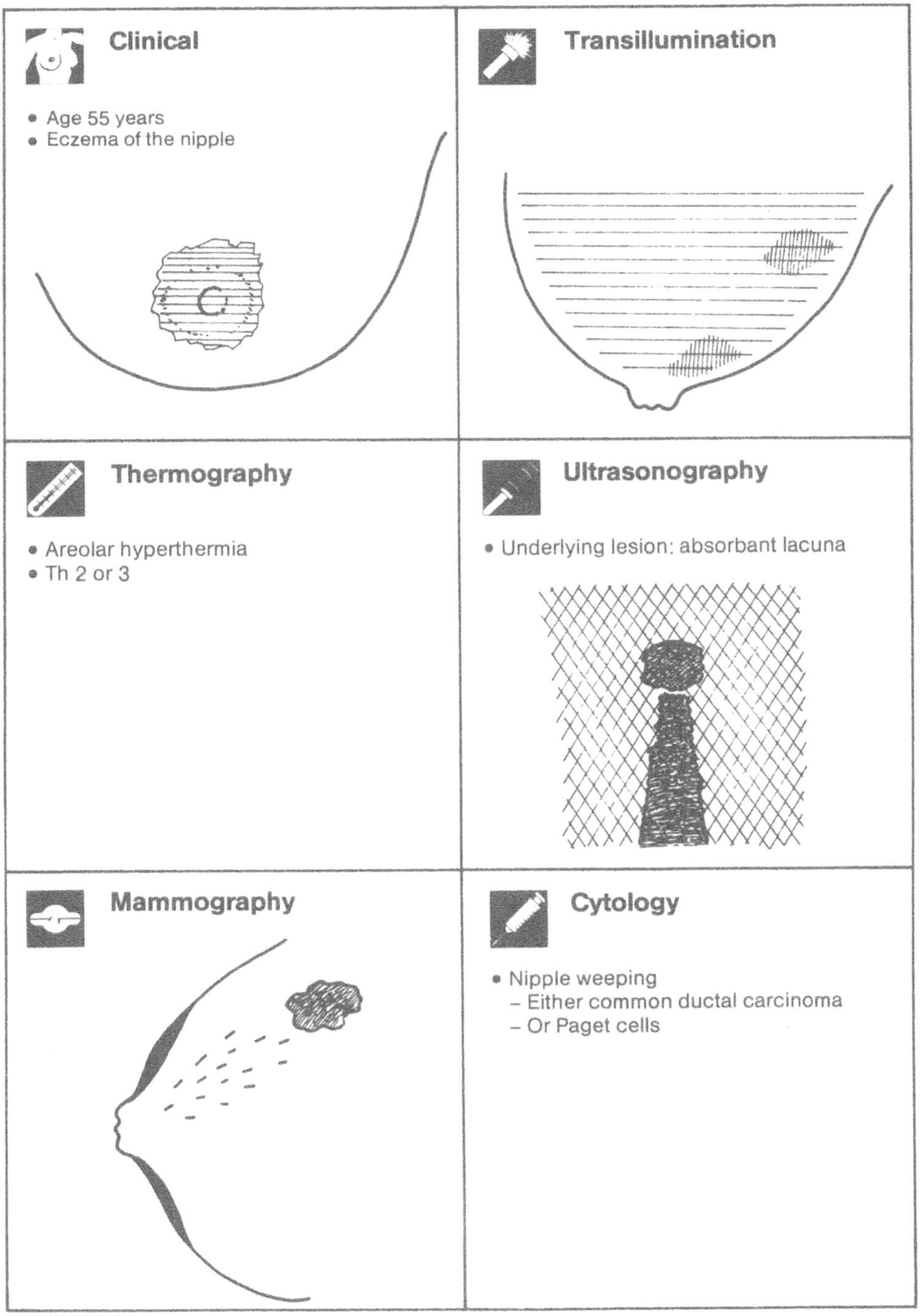

Fig. 139. Paget's disease of the nipple

Clinical

- Hard mass
- Early fixation
- Skin and nipple retraction

Transillumination

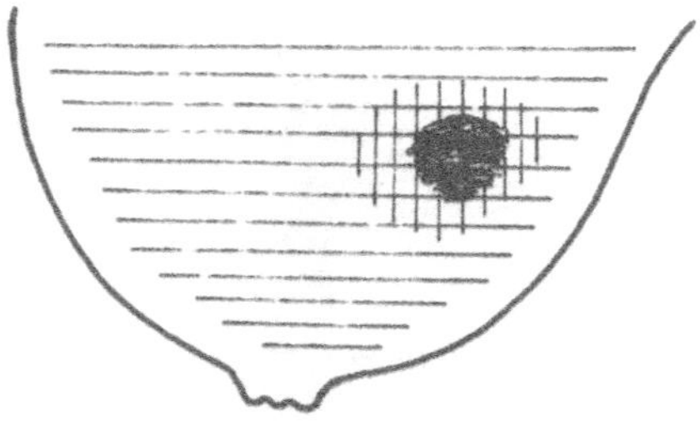

Thermography

- Th ≥ 3

Ultrasonography

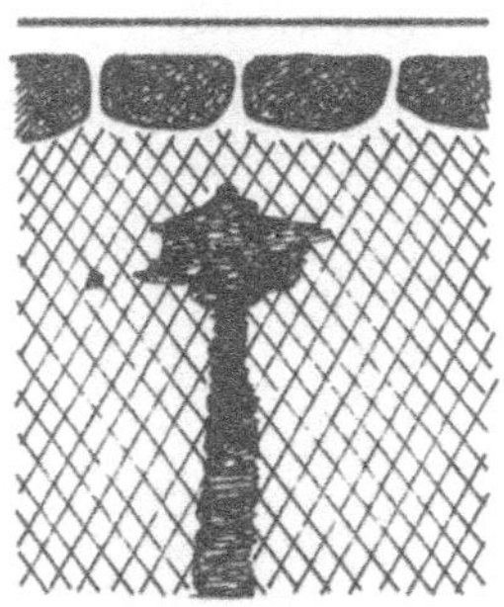

Mammography

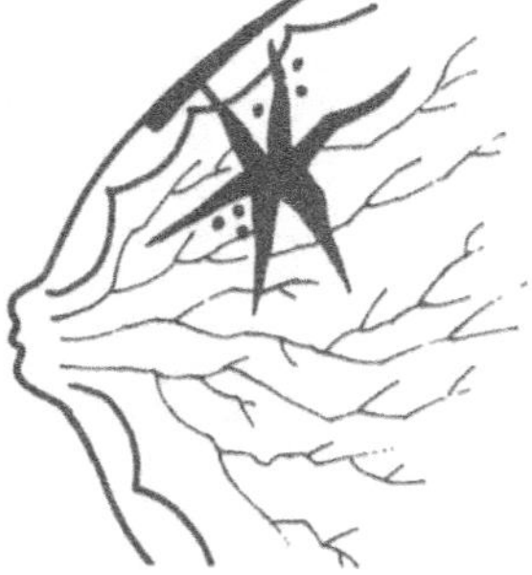

- Radiographic abnormality smaller than the palpated mass

Cytology

- Localization is difficult: risk of false negatives

Fig. 140. Scirrhous carcinoma

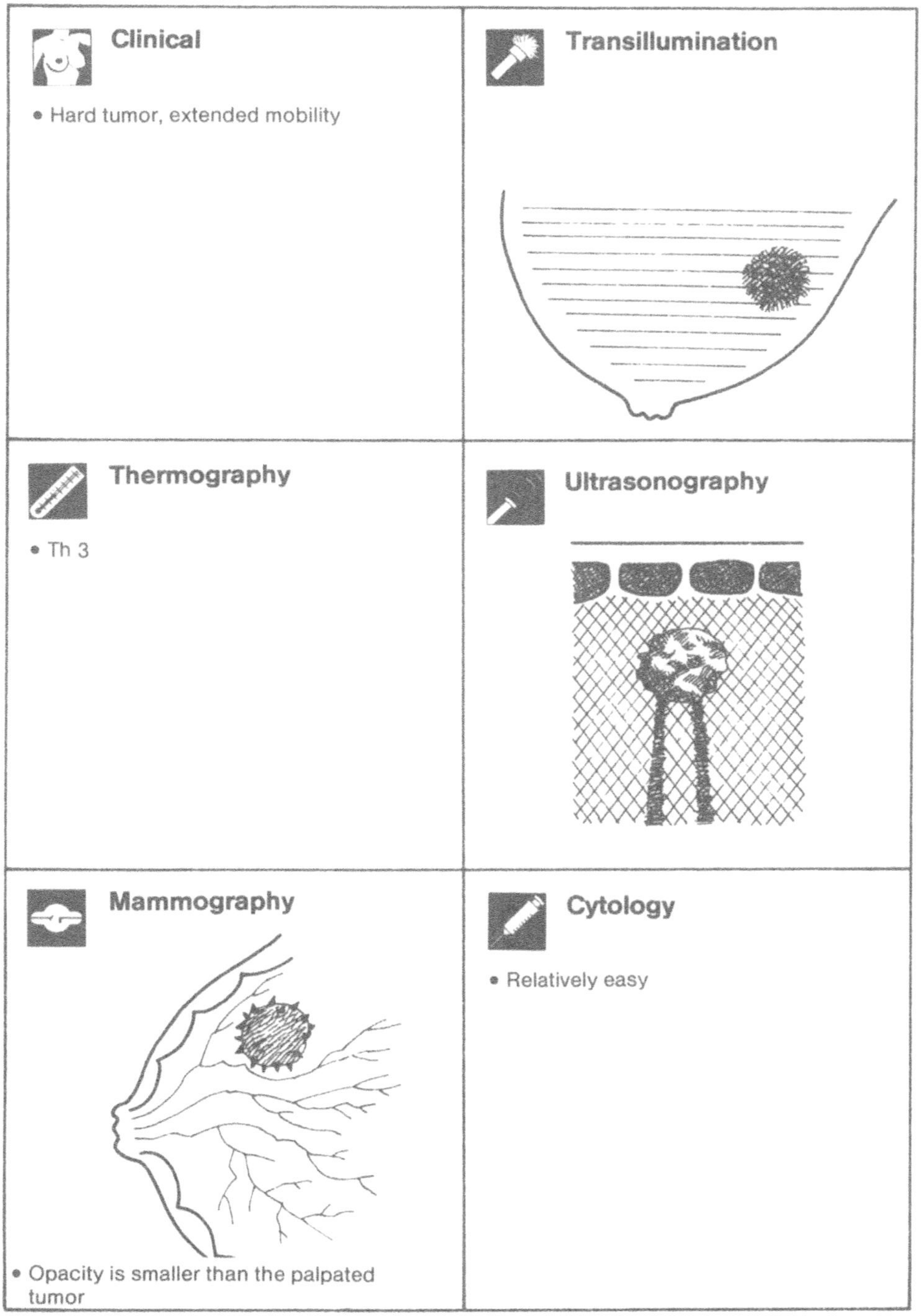

Fig. 141. Nodular carcinoma

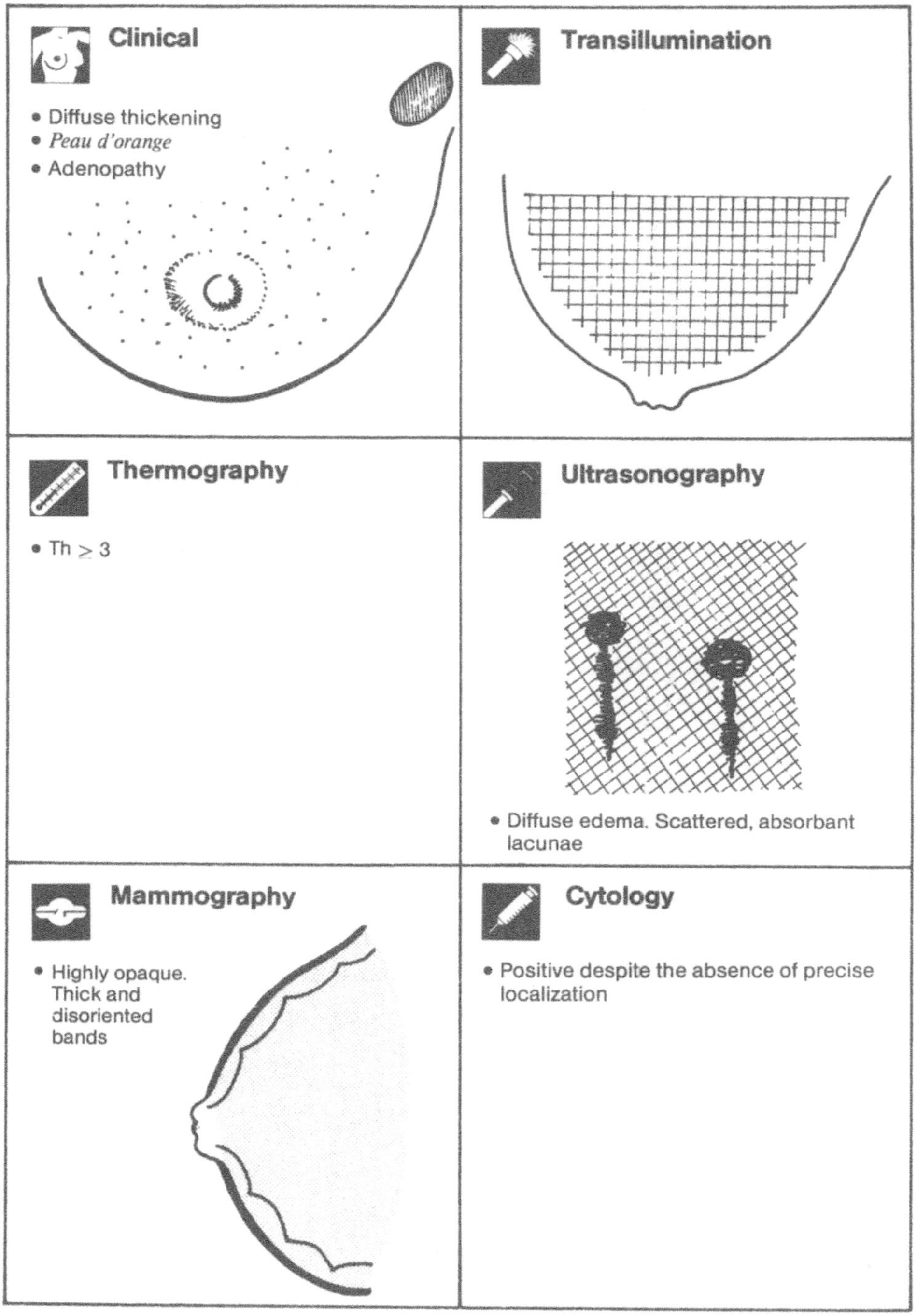

Fig. 142. Diffuse carcinoma

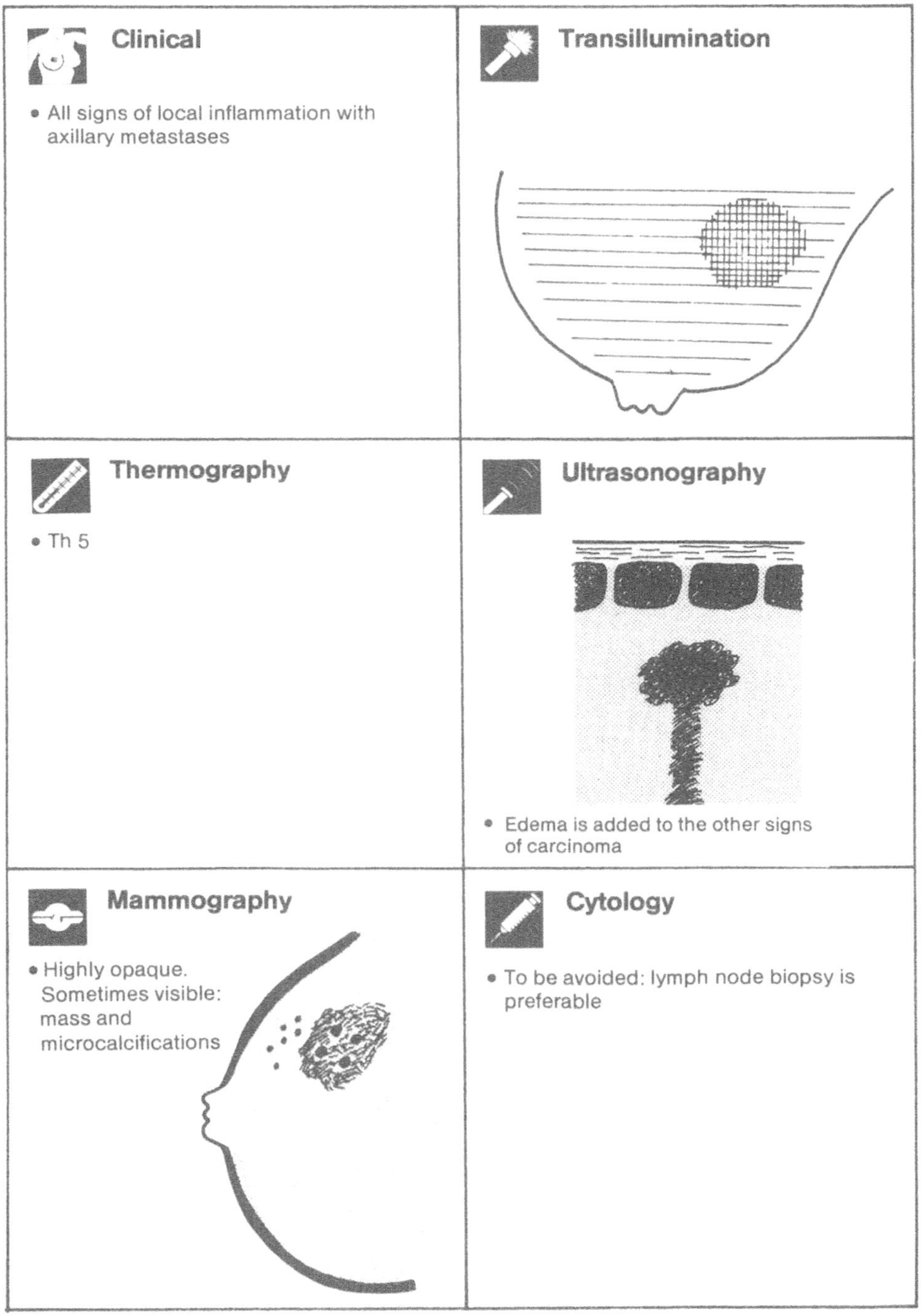

Fig. 143. Inflammatory carcinoma

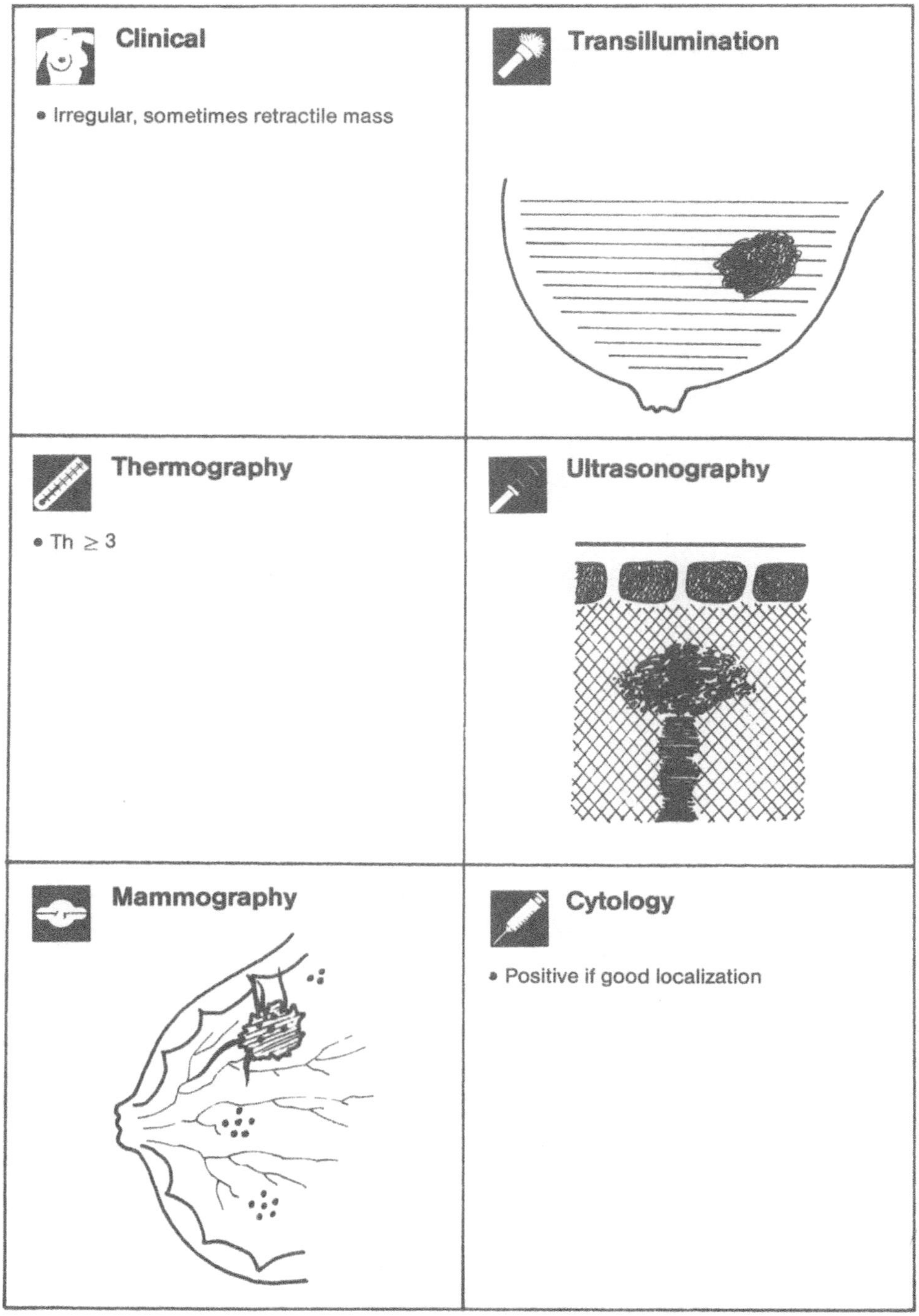

Fig. 144. Invasive lobular carcinoma

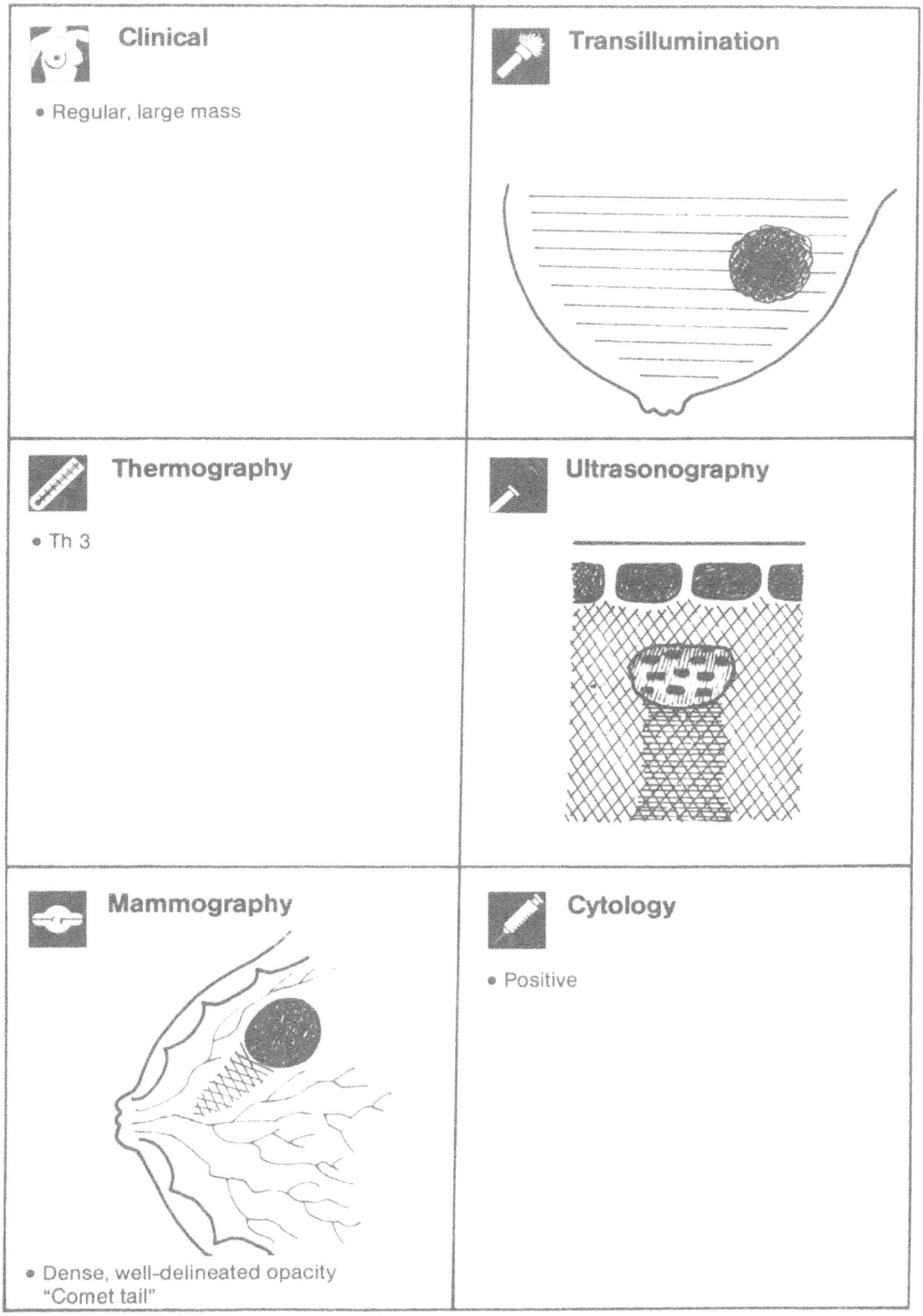

Fig. 145. Medullary carcinoma

Clinical

- Postmenopause
- Firm, resistant, mobile mass

Transillumination

N/A

Thermography

- Th 3

Ultrasonography

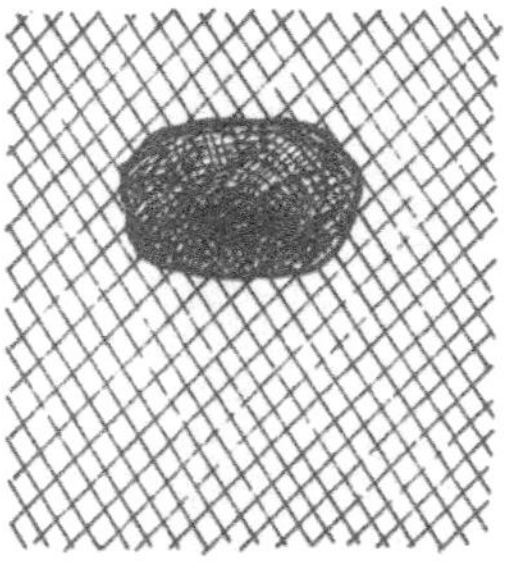

Mammography

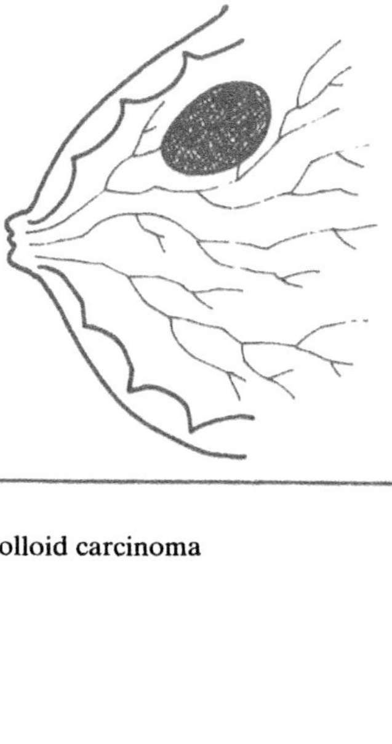

Cytology

- Positive

Fig. 146. Colloid carcinoma

Clinical

- Firm, smooth mass; conserved mobillity

Transillumination

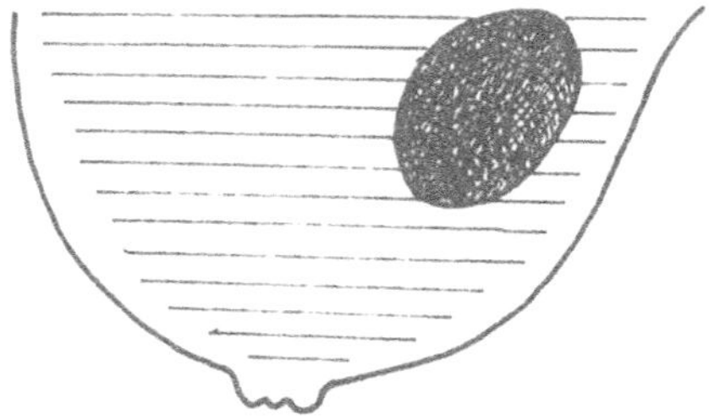

Thermography

- Th ≥ 3

Ultrasonography

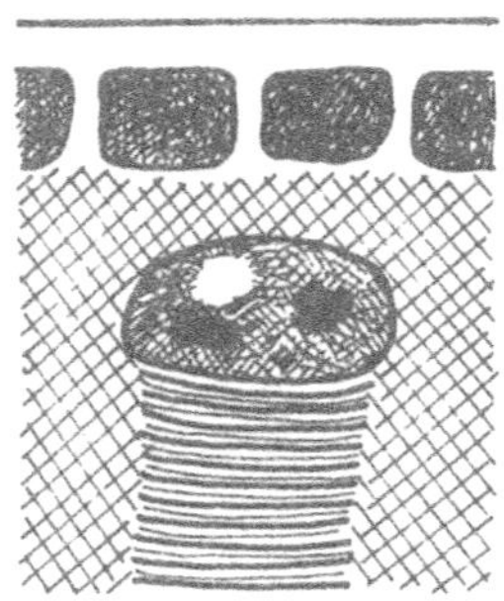

Mammography

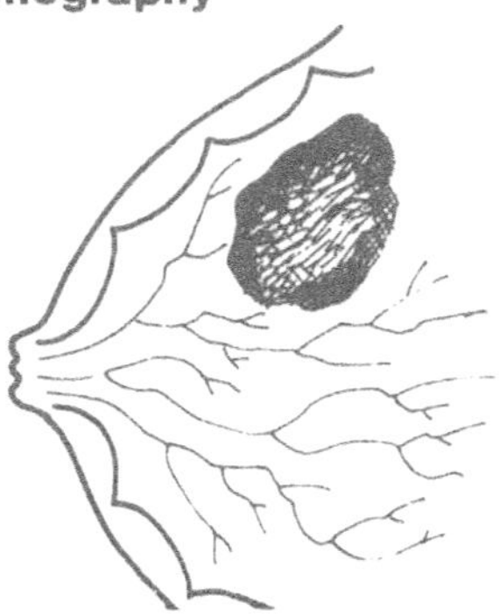

- Dense opacity. Irregular contour
Occasionally special elements (bone)

Cotology

- Histologic examination is necessary to determine type

Fig. 147. Solid sarcoma

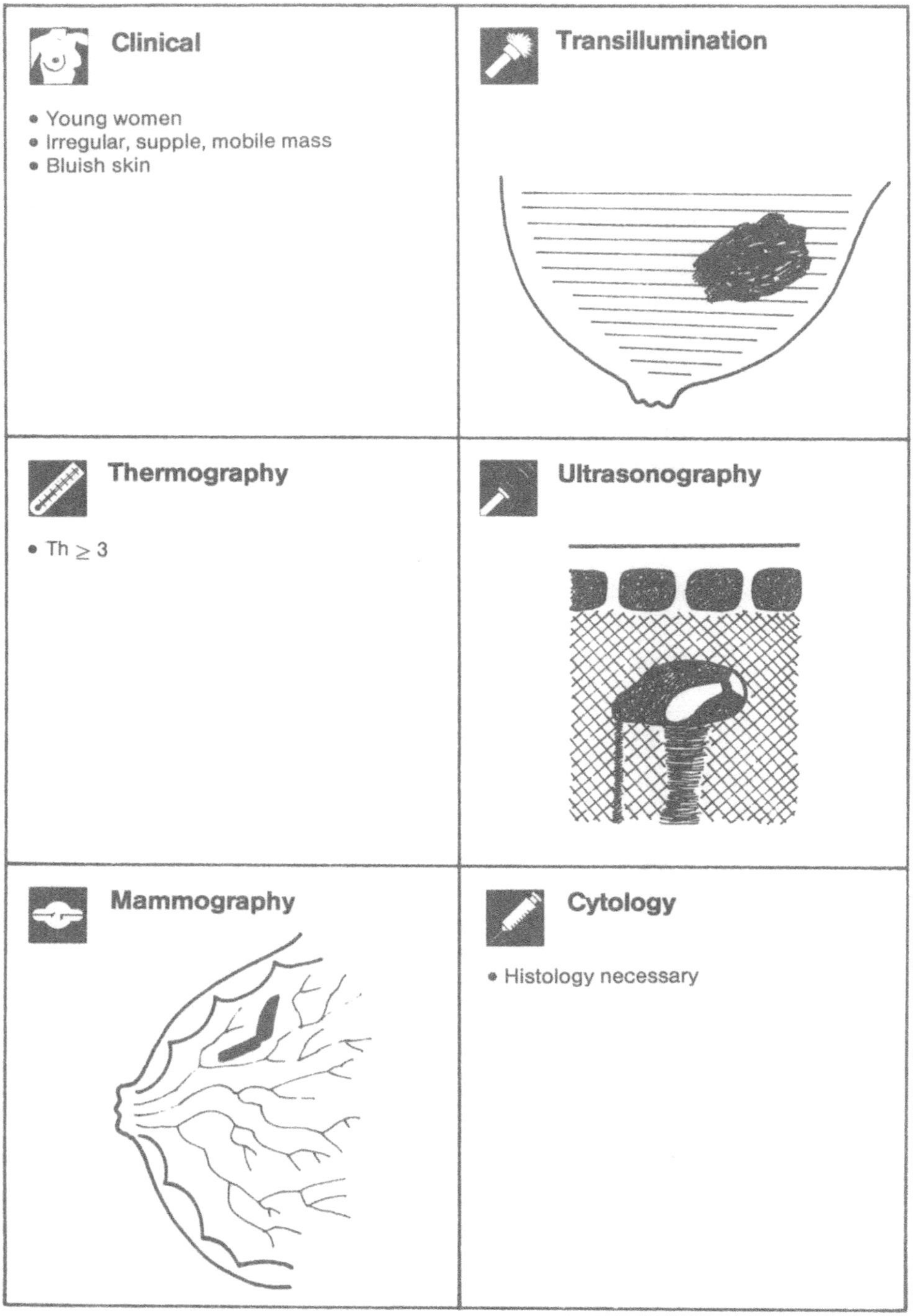

Fig. 148. Hemangioendothelioma

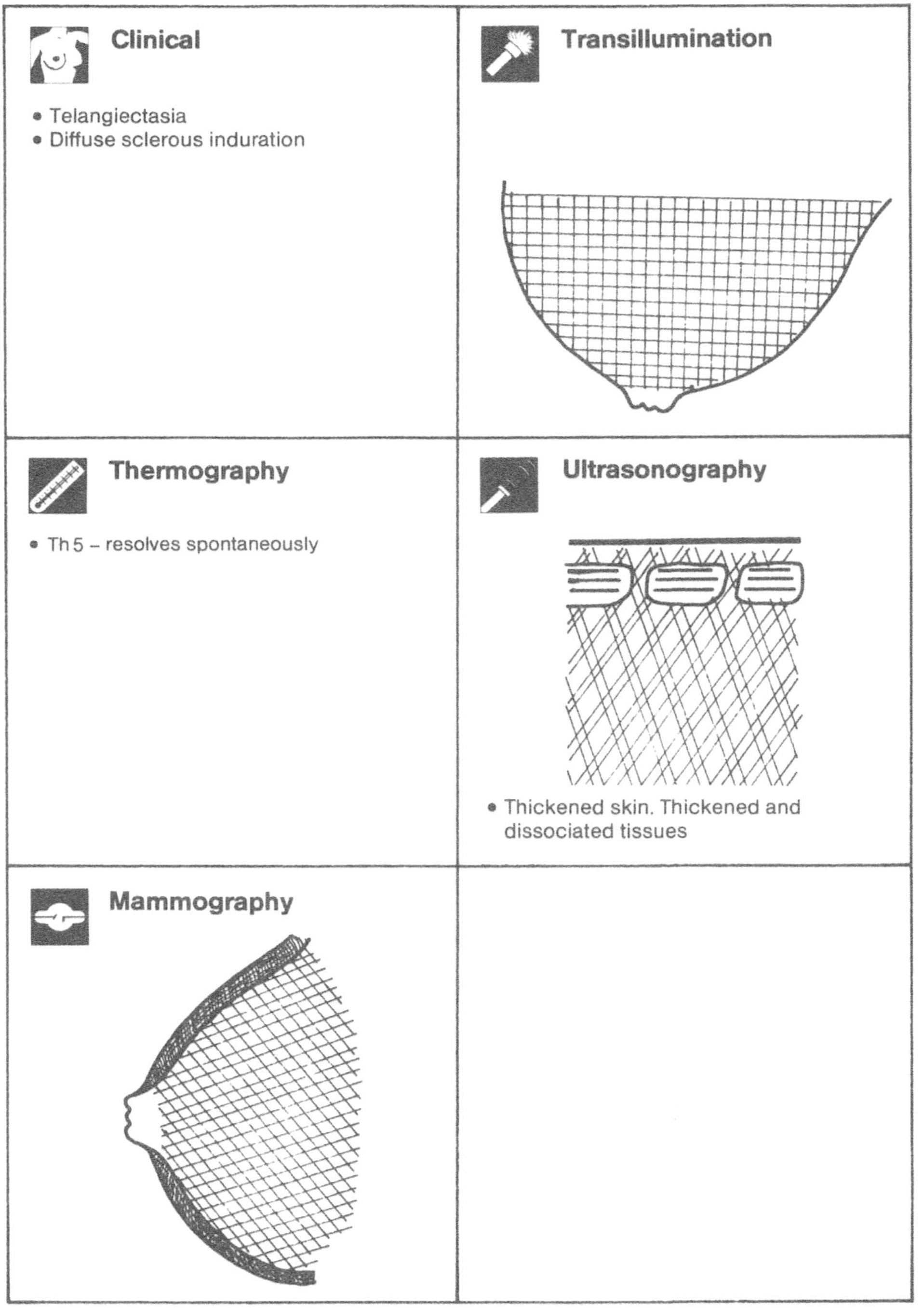

Fig. 149. Irradiated breast

Clinical

- Changeable
- Possible ecchymosis
- Possible mass

Transillumination

- Opaque pool

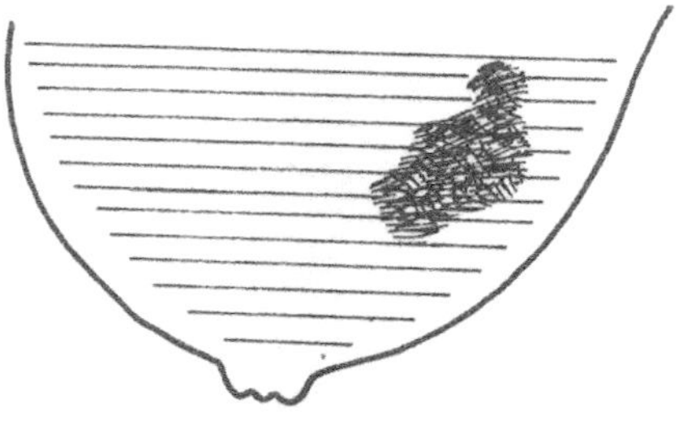

Thermography

N/A

Ultrasonography

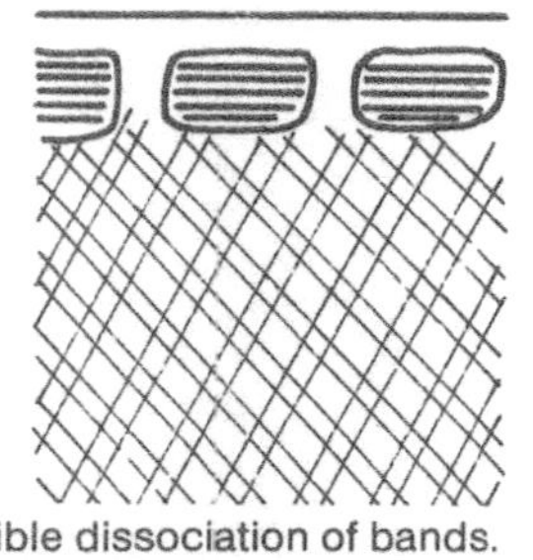

- Possible dissociation of bands. Cutaneous thickening

Mammography

- Possible localized opacity; cutaneous thickening

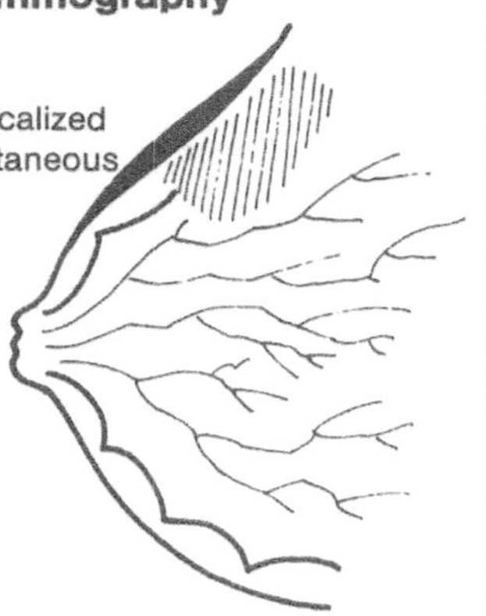

Fig. 150. Hematoma

Clinical

- Resistant nodule

Transillumination

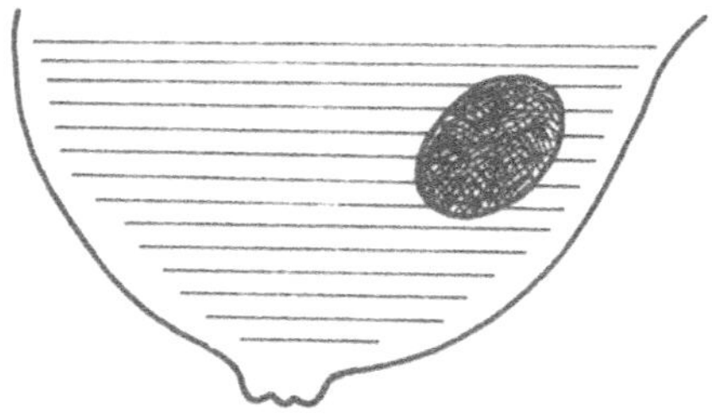

Thermography

N/A

Ultrasonography

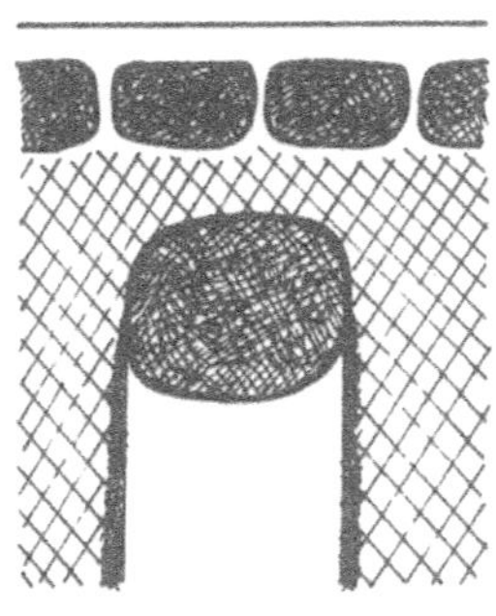

Mammography

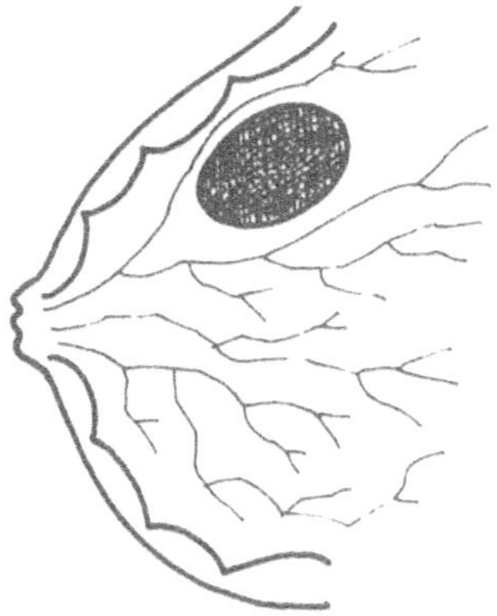

Needle aspiration

- Blood

Fig. 151. Hemorrhagic cyst

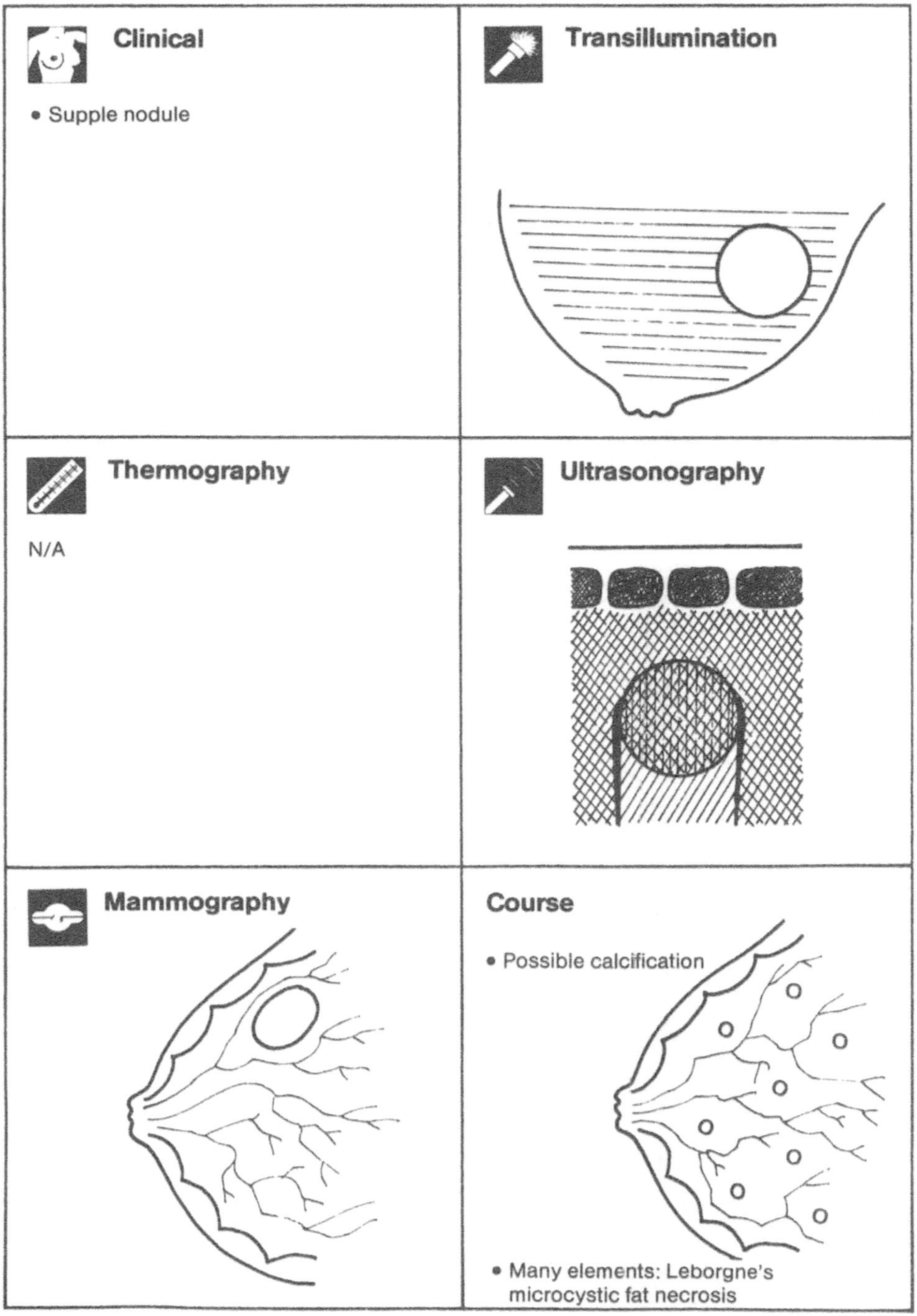

Fig. 152. Fat necrosis (steatonecrosis)

Clinical

- Pain
- Induration
- Skin thickening

Transillumination

N/A

Thermography

N/A

Ultrasonography

- Thickened skin

Mammography

- Thickened skin
- Edematous opacity

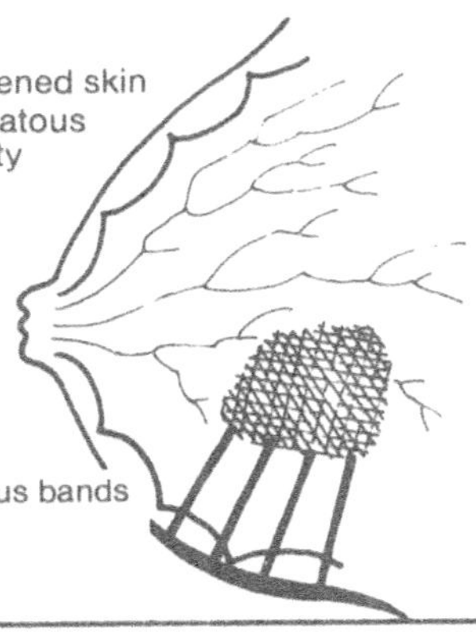

Course

- Resolves
- Fat necrosis
- Calcification

Fig. 153. Microtrauma

Clinical

- Thickened, pink or reddish skin
- Dilated veins
- Mass
- Pain +++

Transillumination

- No characteristic sign

Thermography

- Th $\geq$ 4

Ultrasonography

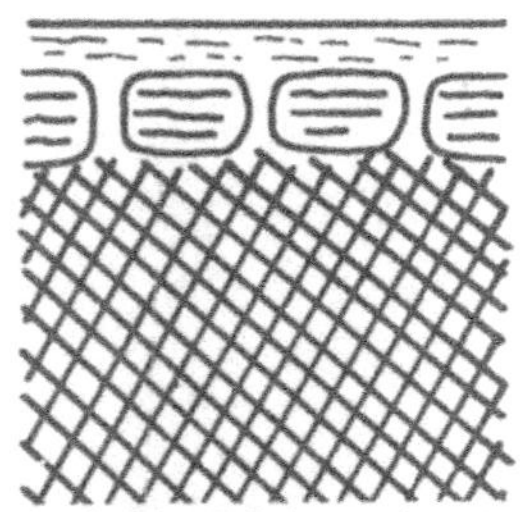

- Thickened skin; thickened and dissociated bands
- Possible primary lesion

Mammography

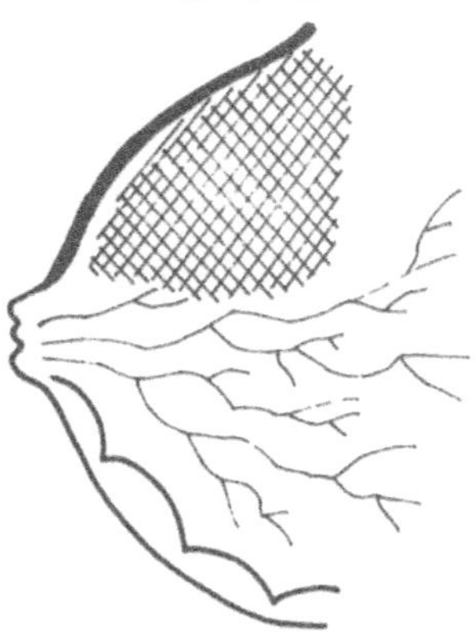

Fig. 154. Acute mastitis

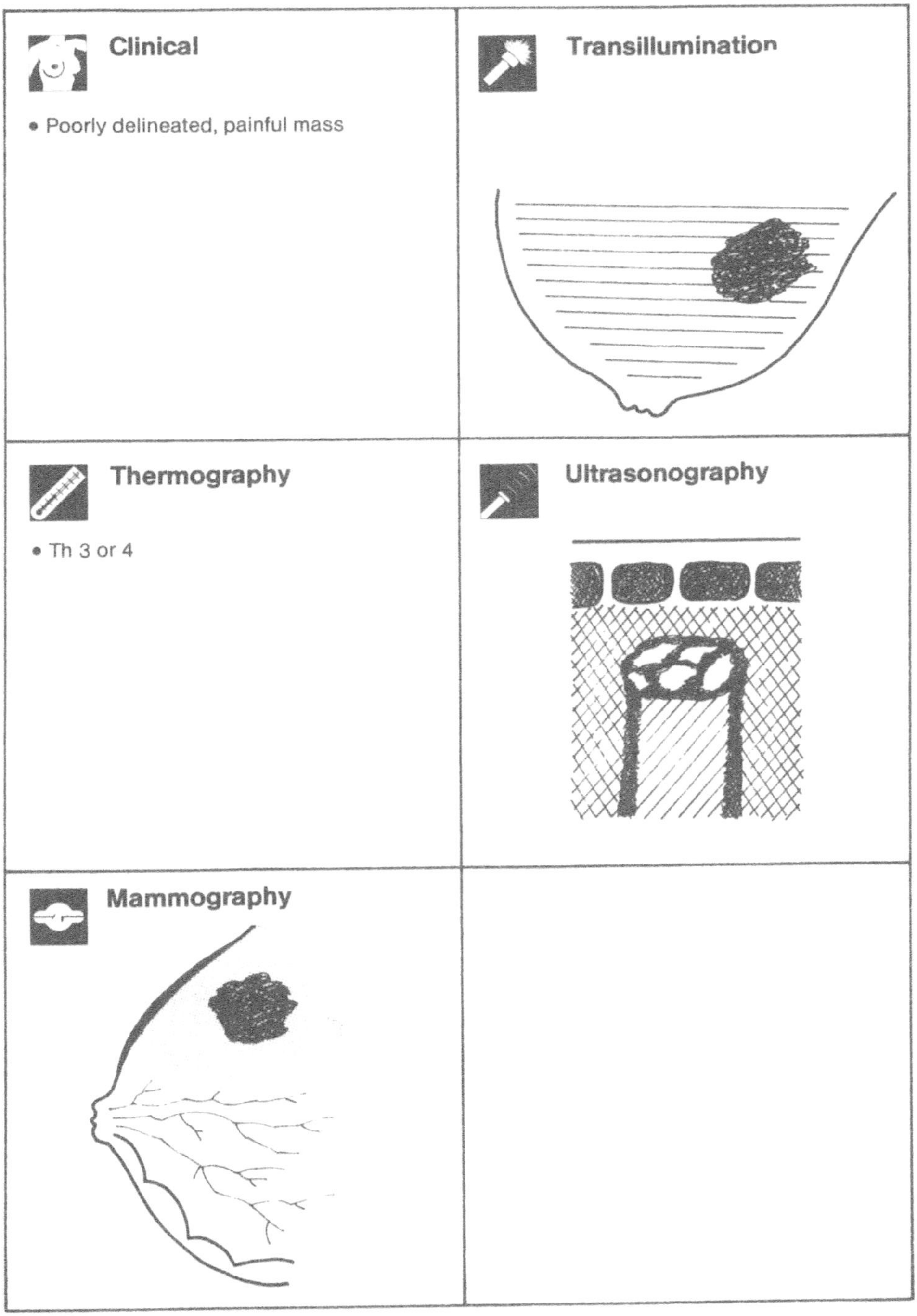

Fig. 155. Abscess

Bibliography

Barnes RB (1967) Thermography-engineering in the practice of medicine. Wiliams & Wilkins, Baltimore, pp 454–465

Basset LW, Gold RH (1982) Mammography, thermography and ultrasound in breast cancer detection. Grune & Stratton, Harcout Brace Jovanovich, New York

Benmussa M, Tristan H (1977) Xérographie mammaire et mammographie. Maloine, Paris

Brux J de (1979) Histopathologie du sein. Masson, Paris

Gros ChM (1963) Les maladies du sein. Masson, Paris

Gros ChM, Sigrist R (1951) La radiographie et la transillumination de la mamelle. Strasbourg Méd Août 1951: 1–15

Haagensen CD (1971) Diseases of the breast, 2nd edn. Saunders, Philadelphia

Hoeffken W, Lanyi M (1977) Mammography. Thieme, Stuttgart

Hollmann KL, Verley JM (1979) Pathologie mammaire. SIMEP, Paris

Hollmann KH, Verley JM (1983) New frontiers in mammary pathology. Plenum Press, New York London

Hubert C (1981) Echographie en pathologie mammaire. Vigot, Paris

Johansson NT (1976) Thermography of the breast. Wien Klin Wochenschr 88(1): 25–29

Lamarque JL (1981) Le sein – Radiodiagnostic clinique. MEDSI, Paris

Leborgne R (1949) Etudes anatomo-radiologiques des tumeurs intracanaliculaires du sein. In: 1er Congrès Uruguayen de Gynécologie, Mars 1949, Montevideo

Lignières B de (1975) Cybernétique hormonale du sein. Senologia 0(1) (Nov 1975): 52–57

Oliva L, Albertis P de (1980) Trattado di senologie. Piccin Editore, Padova

Salomon A (1913) Beiträge zur Pathologie und Klinik der Mammacarcinome. Arch Klin Chir 101: 573–578

Stewart FW (1950) Tumors of the breast. Atlas of tumor pathology. Armed Forces Institute of Pathology, Washington, DC, sect 9–34, p 43

Willemin A (1972) Les images mammographiques. Karger, Basel

Subject Index

GPSR Compliance

The European Union's (EU) General Product Safety Regulation (GPSR) is a set of rules that requires consumer products to be safe and our obligations to ensure this.

If you have any concerns about our products, you can contact us on ProductSafety@springernature.com

In case Publisher is established outside the EU, the EU authorized representative is:

Springer Nature Customer Service Center GmbH
Europaplatz 3
69115 Heidelberg, Germany

Batch number: 10704763

Printed by Printforce, the Netherlands